Low Back Pain Handbook

Low Back Pain Handbook

Edited by

Brian P. D'Orazio, P.T., M.S.

*Clinical Faculty, School of Physical Therapy,
Shenandoah University, Winchester, Virginia;
President, Orthopedic and Sports Physical Therapy
Associates, Inc., Fredericksburg, Virginia*

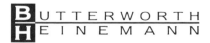

BUTTERWORTH
HEINEMANN

Boston Oxford Johannesburg Melbourne New Delhi Singapore

Every effort has been made to ensure that the drug dosage schedules within this text are accurate and conform to standards accepted at time of publication. However, as treatment recommendations vary in the light of continuing research and clinical experience, the reader is advised to verify drug dosage schedules herein with information found on product information sheets. This is especially true in cases of new or infrequently used drugs.

 Recognizing the importance of preserving what has been written, Butterworth–Heinemann prints its books on acid-free paper whenever possible.

 Butterworth–Heinemann supports the efforts of American Forests and the Global ReLeaf program in its campaign for the betterment of trees, forests, and our environment.

Library of Congress Cataloging-in-Publication Data
D'Orazio, Brian P.
    Low back pain handbook / Brian P. D'Orazio.
        p.   cm.
    Includes bibliographical references and index.
    ISBN 0-7506-9618-4
    1. Backache--Handbooks, manuals, etc. I. Title.
RD771.B217 D67 1999
617.5'64--ddc21
                                98-40679
                                CIP

British Library Cataloguing-in-Publication Data
A catalogue record for this book is available from the British Library.

The publisher offers special discounts on bulk orders of this book.
For information, please contact:

Manager of Special Sales
Butterworth–Heinemann
225 Wildwood Ave.
Woburn, MA 01801-2041
Tel: 781-904-2500
Fax: 781-904-2620

For information on all Butterworth–Heinemann publications available, contact our World Wide Web home page at: http://www.bh.com

10 9 8 7 6 5 4 3 2 1

Printed in the United States of America

Contents

Contributing Authors

Sue E. Curfman, M.S., P.T.
Assistant Professor of Physical Therapy, Shenandoah University, Winchester, Virginia; Affiliate Staff, Winchester Medical Center, Winchester, Virginia

Brian P. D'Orazio, P.T., M.S.
Clinical Faculty, School of Physical Therapy, Shenandoah University, Winchester, Virginia; President, Orthopedic and Sports Physical Therapy Associates, Inc., Fredericksburg, Virginia

Richard Jackson, P.T., O.C.S.
Private Practitioner, Middleburg Physical Therapy, Middleburg, Virginia

Paul L. Lysher, P.T., A.T.C.
Co-Founder and Physical Therapist, Orthopedic and Sports Physical Therapy Associates, Inc., Fredericksburg, Virginia

Marshall A. Rennie, M.P.T.
Physical Therapist, Orthopedic and Sports Physical Therapy Associates, Inc., Fredericksburg, Virginia

Cynthia Burks Starling, M.A.
Pain Management Director, Orthopedic and Sports Physical Therapy Associates, Inc., Fredericksburg, Virginia

Caroline Tritsch, M.P.T.
Physical Therapist, Orthopedic and Sports Physical Therapy Associates, Inc., Fredericksburg, Virginia

Shane A. Vath, M.P.T.
Assistant Department Head and Staff Physical Therapist, Naval Medical Clinic–Quantico, United States Navy, Quantico, Virginia

Preface

The purpose of *Low Back Pain Handbook* is to provide students and clinicians with information on the low back, not just the lumbar spine, and to do so in a user-friendly format. The format of this book, as the title implies, is intended to be as close to a handbook as biomedical and clinical science allow. At some point in the distant future, a handbook on low back pain (LBP) filled with menus of specific treatments dealing with specific categories of problems will be written. These treatments will have been scientifically measured for effectiveness, and clinicians will be able to rely on that information to guide treatment. This text, it is hoped, is a step in that direction. The information in each chapter is scientifically validated as well as possible, and yet, many of the strategies still rely on a good deal of clinical art.

The intent of each chapter in *Low Back Pain Handbook* is to provide readily usable tools for clinical treatment, measurement of outcomes, and rehabilitation protocols. This text covers three broad categories: anatomy and etiology, evaluation, and management. The information in each section is as simplified, structured, and visual as possible. There is no pretense that each section is comprehensive; however, the pages do provide the information necessary to improve clinical competence. *Low Back Pain Handbook* is applicable to multiple disciplines, as evidenced in Chapter 1, which uniquely integrates anatomy with patient evaluation. The final chapters of the text are specifically for physical therapists, but general knowledge of this information is important for surgeons who are active participants in the process of recommending rehabilitation strategies for specific surgical procedures.

The goal of Chapter 1 is to integrate a somewhat dry science, anatomy, with the clinical science of evaluation. The reader should enjoy the author's weaving of the two topics, creating a clinically oriented anatomy chapter with clear illustrations and a strong emphasis on the biomechanics of function. An investigation into LBP etiology always includes a thorough examination of anatomy, and it is from that examination that logically sequenced treatment is conceived.

Although LBP in most patients has a musculoskeletal origin, Chapter 2 examines the influence of diseases and disorders on the presentation of LBP. Recognizing that a disease process or disorder may be at work in the patient's LBP complaint is the first step in investigating a potentially critical health issue. Also included in this chapter is information on typical referral patterns from organ systems.

The first step in evaluating a patient's LBP comes from a basic examination of his or her medical, social, psychological, and work history. Chapter 3 begins Section II by discussing the logic and necessity of taking a thorough history and also provides the forms necessary to complete a patient's history. Specific systems-review forms allow a clinician to more thoroughly explore areas such as the urogenital system.

Assessment of patients with LBP should begin with a thorough biomechanical evaluation. For patients with musculoskeletal LBP, the amelioration of aberrant biomechanical variables can be critical to resolving symptoms. A leg length discrepancy, once thought to be of no consequence, is an example of a biomechanical dysfunction that has been demonstrated to correlate highly with complaints of LBP. The considerable scientific information in Chapter 4 regarding biomechanical influences on LBP allows clinicians to better understand how abnormal alignment or movement may contribute to LBP and how variables as far away as the foot can influence the pelvis and lumbar spine.

Chapters 5–7 explore patient management, beginning with an examination of the multiple factors that modulate a patient's response and concluding with postsurgical protocols in Chapter 7. Chapter 5 examines the complex interrelationships between a patient's perception of his or her pain and how this relates to disability. The complex relationships between pain and disability are often the reasons that good treatment techniques fail. Psychosocial events can produce barriers to recovery that unwittingly undermine disability resolution. In Chapter 5, examination of psychosocial management strategies is aided by the use of disability measurement tools. These forms will help clinicians identify how patients perceive their disability and when this perception may be out of proportion with their impairment. Chapter 5 also offers treatment strategies that decrease the difference between the patient's disability and his or her measured impairment.

With research consistently indicating that exercise is the best treatment for most types of LBP, research for the prescription of exercise has been limited. To prescribe, clinicians must be able to classify. The process of classifying patients with LBP is controversial and evolving. Chapter 6 presents a basic rationale for patient classification that translates knowledge gained from evaluation of neuromotor control into the prescription of meaningful rehabilitation programs.

The final chapter, Chapter 7, examines postsurgical rehabilitation, an area in which there is a surprising paucity of information. The prescription of rehabilitation for patients who have undergone a lumbar surgical procedure has largely relied on the patient's report of symptoms to guide treatment. Symptoms, however, are only one dimension of a complex evaluative system that includes physiologic healing rates, biomechanical stresses, socioeconomic issues, and longitudinal outcome studies. This chapter is one of the first to establish specific temporal guidelines for postsurgical rehabilitation. These temporal guidelines are based on an evolving body of knowledge, along with recommendations by experts in the field.

New approaches to the treatment of LBP have been offered for centuries. Many of these approaches parallel either new scientific discoveries or new philosophies about the origins of LBP. Even today, new treatment techniques are offered in courses that are, at best, speculative. As Rothstein states, "Some people would have you believe that they have the secret recipe—treatments they have discovered, management protocols they are marketing, or techniques they are willing to teach—but such people are masters of the evidence-free argument."* As LBP research advances, all clinicians can look forward to validated treatment techniques and performance measures that are accurate prognosticators of treatment outcomes. *Low Back Pain Handbook* has carefully integrated a vast scientific database into a user-friendly format that provides a scientifically refined clinical art. With advances in research over the past two decades, a basic curriculum of information now exists that, when followed, offers many patients today with a considerably more efficacious resolution to their disability.

In the coming decade, research will continue to expand in the direction of defining causative agents for LBP, while testing classification systems that will further outcomes research. Although debates will remain about the efficacy of specific approaches, a basic approach to rehabilitation will crystallize. Even with a clearer view of efficacious rehabilitation approaches, mastery of this basic information on LBP is and will remain a daunting pursuit for years to come. The clinical approaches presented in *Low Back Pain Handbook* reflect the science of LBP research, synthesized and refined to yield rehabilitation strategies that will lead clinicians into the twenty-first century.

---

*Rothstein JM. Editor's note to physical therapy. J Am Phys Ther Assoc 1998;78(7):676.

Low Back Pain Handbook

1

Anatomic Applications to Evaluating Patients with Low Back Pain

Sue E. Curfman

What are the normal three-dimensional relationships of the bony elements of the low back? What structures are innervated and are therefore potential sources of pain? What structures are the sources of your patient's pain? What structures are biomechanical causes of dysfunction? What is the relationship of the morphology of a structure and its function or dysfunction? How would foreshortening of these structures affect your patient's function? How would foreshortening or lengthening of these structures present during your clinical examination? What exactly are you palpating when your hands are placed in a certain location? What structures are abnormally lengthened given that your patient has this postural abnormality? How can you test this? Is this structure malleable and hence will you be able to correct your patient's posture? What structures are you stressing during your clinical examination? Answering these types of questions necessitates a working knowledge of the anatomy of the low back. Unless structure is understood, identifying the relationships between signs and symptoms and movement will be guesswork at best.

This chapter describes the anatomic structures and relationships of the low back in order to facilitate a greater appreciation of the examination procedure, the findings, and, ultimately, the treatment of patients with low back pain (LBP). Appendix 1-1, at the end of this chapter, presents these structures visually. The low back is operationally defined as the area between T12 and the hips. Thus the joints included are the facet joints (also called *zygapophyseal* or *posterior intervertebral joints*), the intervertebral joints (also called *anterior intervertebral joints*), the sacroiliac joints, the pubic symphysis, and the hip joints. If we obtain satisfactory results with a patient yet lack a thorough understanding of what structures we were actually influencing and why our treatments were effective, we are less likely to replicate these results with another patient. If this is the case, patient evaluation and treatment is reduced to trial and error. A thorough understanding of the structures that are the sources of pain and dysfunction is critical.

A thorough description and review of a comprehensive evaluation procedure for the low back is beyond the scope of this chapter. Rather, the chapter describes general categories of evaluation and integrates the anatomy being studied within each of these categories. See the chapters that follow for a more comprehensive discussion of evaluation procedures.

Anatomic Features on Visual Inspection

A working knowledge of anatomy is compulsory during visual inspection. As the clinician observes the patient, he or she should be able to see with a "mind's eye" the structures that are located deep to the skin and the three-dimensional relationships among these structures. The first step in identifying potential problems within more deeply located structures is visual inspection. The surface anatomy is first examined during the visual inspection of the patient. Inspection of the general body type, symmetry of bony elements and soft tissues, condition of the skin, and alignment of the body in general and spinal alignment more specifically is typically performed during the visual inspection of a patient.

Body Type

The anatomic features indicated by observing body type typically include the general bony architecture, muscle mass, and the presence of adipose tissue. Body types are divided into three categories: ectomorph, mesomorph, and endomorph. The ectomorphic body type is characterized by a predominance of tissues derived from the ectoderm, which is the outer layer of cells of the developing embryo. Linearity of body build with sparse muscular development is characteristic of individuals classified as ectomorphic. The mesomorphic body type is characterized by a predominance of tissues derived from the mesoderm, which is the middle layer of the developing embryo. The mesoderm gives rise to connective, muscular, and skeletal tissues in addition to other tissues. Typically, a mesomorph is a well proportioned individual. The endomorphic body type is characterized by a predominance of tissues derived from the endoderm, the inner cellular layer of the embryo. Typically these individuals have a higher percentage of body fat. It is important to note the distribution of adipose tissue because adipose tissue is innervated and hence a potential source of pain. The importance of noting body types lies in the ability to identify the biomechanical stress created when an individual participates in a given activity. Body type has an effect on how an individual will handle biomechanical stresses.

Symmetry of Bony Elements

The frontal plane relationships (Figure 1A-1) typically include the height of the shoulders, pelvis, hips, knees, and ankles and the position of the scapula. In the sagittal plane, the relationships of the head to the trunk, the shoulders to the thorax, the pelvis to the trunk, and the lower extremity joints to each other are all considered (Figure 1A-2). The rotational positions of the body are observed during the visual inspection of the transverse plane relationships. Asymmetry of the rotation of the head on the trunk, the pelvis on the lower extremity, and the leg on the foot/ankle may all be considered here.

Evaluation of Active Low Back Movements

Structures that both create and limit motion assist in the production of movement. As dynamic structures, skeletal muscles are the obvious movers of the low back. Noncontractile connective tissues such as the ligaments, fascia, capsules, and discs guide and limit movement. The bony configurations of the spine, hips, and pelvis also play a major role in low back movement. Muscles, although viewed primarily as dynamic structures because of their contractile elements, also have a static role and hence provide stability.

Muscles

A detailed description of the attachments and actions of each of the spinal movers will not be provided in the body of this chapter. Refer to Appendix 1-2, found at the end of this chapter, for detailed information on each muscle influencing the trunk.

In general, the muscles of the lumbar spine can be divided into five major groups: (1) the superficial muscles of the back, (2) the erector spinae group, (3) the transversospinalis group, (4) the muscles of the anterior abdominal wall, and (5) the muscles of the posterior abdominal wall. Any muscle crossing the spine but not necessarily attaching to the spine may create motion at the spine and may alter the alignment of the spine. Any muscle crossing joints of the spine is able to produce force at these joints and thus must be considered in the evaluation of the spine.

Making the evaluation of the low back even more complex is the fact that muscles not crossing the lumbar spine but influencing the position of the pelvis must also be considered. Any muscle attaching to the innominate bone can alter the position of the innominate bone and hence the position of the lumbar spine. Therefore, all muscles in the three compartments of the thigh that attach to the innominate bone must be considered in the evaluation of the low back. Because the lumbar spine allows movement in all three cardinal planes to varying degrees, muscles producing osteokinematic effects in all three planes will be addressed here. The muscles of the hip and thigh that affect the spine will be subsequently presented.

Extensors of the Lumbar Spine
The muscles active during lumbar extension include those in the erector spinae, the transversospinalis, and the superficial back muscle groups. The superficial muscles of the low back are not innervated by dorsal rami and thus are not considered true back muscles. The muscles in the superficial low back group are the latissimus dorsi and the lower trapezius (Figure 1A-3). Because each of these muscles attaches to the dorsal spine, they can influence the movement and position of the spine into extension. The true back muscles include the muscles in the erector spinae group and the transversospinalis group. The erector spinae muscle group, specifically the spinalis thoracis, longissimus thoracis, and iliocostalis lumborum subgroups, produce extension of the lumbar and lower thoracic spines (Figure 1A-4). While the transversospinalis group primarily serves other functions, the fact that it is located posterior to the spine indicates a role in spinal extension. Included in this transversospinalis group are the semispinalis, multifidus, and rotatores (Figure 1A-5). The multifidus is the only muscle of this group that is significantly developed in the lumbar region (Figure 1A-6). Figure 1A-7 demonstrates the three-dimensional relationships of the musculature of the thoracic spine. Figure 1A-8 demonstrates the three-dimensional relationships of the lumbar musculature.

Flexors of the Lumbar Spine
Generally, muscles that flex the spine are located anterior to the spine. Included in this functional group are the rectus abdominus and the external and internal abdominal obliques (Figure 1A-9). The psoas major, attaching to the bodies, discs, and transverse processes of the lumbar spine, is a muscle of the posterior abdominal wall (Figure 1A-10). It is said by some to produce lumbar flexion, as in raising the trunk from the recumbent position.[1] Others suggest that the psoas major muscle can act as either a flexor or an extensor of the lumbar spine (WJ Personius, personal communication,

1993). Personius hypothesized that because some fibers of the psoas major course anterior and others posterior to the instantaneous axis of rotation of the lumbar motion segments, the psoas may respectively flex and extend the lumbar spine (Figure 1A-11). Another hypothesis is that the psoas major may act as an extensor of the upper and a flexor of the lower lumbar motion segments. Lordosis could be operationalized as flexion of the lower lumbar motion segments and extension of the upper lumbar motion segments, similar to the position noted with forward head posture. This hypothesis is supported by the fact that a greater number of psoas major fibers cross posterior to the axes of the upper lumbar segments and anterior to the axes of the lower lumbar segments. Without dispute, the psoas major crosses over lumbar spine joints and is capable of creating joint forces. It must be considered when examining the lumbar spine.

Lateral Flexors of the Lumbar Spine

Those muscles most capable of producing lateral flexion of the spine are located farthest away from the midline (Figures 1A-12, 1A-13, 1A-14). Therefore, the iliocostalis lumborum, iliocostalis thoracis, the external and internal abdominal obliques, and the quadratus lumborum are the major muscles providing lateral flexion of the spine. The transversospinalis group, the medial erector spinae muscles, the rectus abdominus, and the psoas major muscles are not major contributors to lateral flexion of the spine because they are more medially located.

Rotators of the Lumbar Spine

Although the lumbar spine allows little rotation because of its bony configuration, it remains important to consider the muscles capable of producing a rotational moment through it. Although these muscles do not create a large degree of segmental rotation, they are capable of producing joint forces and may limit normal arthrokinematic movements. Limited segmental arthrokinematic movements may lead to losses in spinal range of motion produced in any plane. The multifidus is capable of producing lumbar rotation, given the superomedial fiber direction (Figure 1A-15). *Gray's Anatomy*[1] states that the multifidus and other short dorsal muscles are primarily stabilizers of the spine. The internal and external abdominal oblique muscles are the muscles most capable of producing rotation in the lumbar spine (see Figure 1A-9).

Muscles Moving the Pelvis

Pelvic motion creates motion in the lumbar spine. Muscles that attach to the pelvis may create secondary lumbar movements. The muscles crossing the spine and attaching to the innominate bone are the latissimus dorsi, the iliocostalis lumborum, the quadratus lumborum, and the abdominals. These muscles directly create motion of the lumbar spine.

Another category of muscles needs to be considered as potential movers of the lumbar spine. These muscles do not cross the spine but attach to the innominate bone. This set of muscles creates indirect lumbar movement. It includes the sartorius and rectus femoris from the anterior compartment of the thigh (Figure 1A-16); the semimembranosus, semitendinosus, and the long head of the biceps femoris from the posterior compartment of the thigh (Figure 1A-17); and all of the muscles in the medial compartment of the thigh, including the gracilis, pectineus, adductor brevis, adductor longus, and adductor magnus (Figure 1A-18). The muscles of the buttock also attach to the innominate and so can have an effect on lumbar spine movement (Figure 1A-19). The muscles of the buttock region include the gluteus maximus, gluteus medius, and gluteus minimus and the tensor fascia lata. The gluteus maximus, because of its attachment to the fascia of the erector spinae and to the sacrum, has an additional effect on the lumbar spine and may pull the sacrum posteriorly, as can the multifidus. The external rotators of the hip, the piriformis, the gemellus superior, the obturator internus, the gemellus inferior, the obturator externus, and the quadratus femoris, located deep within the buttock, also attach to the innominate and/or sacrum and thus potentially move the pelvis on the lumbar spine. In light of the attachment of the piriformis to the ventral surface of the sacrum, the piriformis may pull the sacrum anteriorly. Generally, anterior thigh muscles increase lumbar lordosis by anteriorly tilting the pelvis. Posterior thigh muscles posteriorly tilt the pelvis, decreasing lumbar lordosis (Figure 1A-20). Foreshortened medial thigh muscles lower the contralateral pelvis, while the buttock muscles, if foreshortened, raise the contralateral pelvis.

Bony Limiters of Movement

In addition to the muscles of the spine, the bony configuration of the spine acts to guide movements. According to data obtained by White and Panjabi[2] (Figure 1A-21), the amount of spinal movements is variable depending on the direction moved. This is largely a result of the orientation of the facet joints. The lumbar facet joints are oriented 90 degrees up from the transverse plane and 45 degrees from the sagittal plane (Figures 1A-22, 1A-23). More specifically, the upper lumbar facet joints are primarily oriented in the sagittal plane with the most anterior aspect of the joint surface located in the frontal plane. These facets are said to be J shaped. In the lower lumbar spine, the facets more closely resemble the letter C. In these lower segments, greater anterior-posterior translation can occur in the absence of the portion of the facet joint located in the frontal plane (Figure 1A-24). For this reason, the lower lumbar motion segments allow greater degrees of flexion and extension compared with the upper lumbar segments. Lumbar sagittal plane motion exceeds frontal or transverse plane motion. The motion segments of T12–L1 and L1–L2 allow 12 degrees of combined flexion and extension each. L2–L3 allows 14 degrees combined flexion and extension. Inferior to L2–L3 the combined flexion and extension available at each of the motion segments increases by 1 degree. L5–S1 offers the greatest combined flexion and extension at 17 degrees. In general, the amount of available flexion and extension increases as one descends the lumbar spine.

Lumbar lateral flexion is greatest in the mid-lumbar motion segments, averaging 6–8 degrees, and least at the L5–S1 motion segment, with only 3 degrees. Rotation is the most limited osteokinematic factor in the lumbar spine. In comparison to the average of 8–9 degrees of rotation available in the lower thoracic motion segments, the lumbar motion segments provide 1–2 degrees of motion, with L5–S1 being most restricted.

The configuration of the facets of the T12 vertebra is also a factor that guides lumbar motion. The superior articular facets of T12 are oriented generally like those of the thoracic spine, 60 degrees up from the transverse plane and 20 degrees out from the frontal plane. The inferior articular facet of T12 is oriented similar to the lumbar facets, and therefore this segment is known as a transitional segment. Assuming normal posture, the line of gravity falls through the transitional segments, indicating the transition from thoracic kyphosis to lumbar lordosis. Movements may be limited at this segment because of the differences in the superior and inferior facet orientations.

Anatomic Features in a Neurologic Evaluation

Because of the nervous system's relationship with the spine, it is imperative that a broad neurologic evaluation be performed when examining a patient with LBP. Because neural tissue is susceptible to pressure, any location in which a neural structure is located within a relatively confined space, bony or otherwise, is a potential source for a space-occupying lesion. The spinal cord and cauda equina located within the spinal canal and the spinal nerves located within the intervertebral foramina are examples of areas in which there is a potential for space-occupying lesions. Similarly, neural tissue may be susceptible to pressure from soft tissues such as muscular foreshortening, inflammation, or connective tissue restrictions. What would the signs and symptoms be if a patient had an impingement of neural tissue? What evaluation procedures are necessary to rule out neurologic involvement con-

Table 1-1 Lower Extremity Deep Tendon Reflexes

Reflex	Muscle group	Root levels tested
Knee jerk	Quadriceps	L3–L4
Ankle jerk	Gastrocnemius and soleus	S1–S2

current with your patient's LBP? Examination procedures conducted to evaluate nervous system function may include, but are not limited to, deep tendon reflexes (DTRs), lower extremity strength and sensory assessments, and special tests, such as the straight leg raise, slump, and neural tension tests.

Deep Tendon Reflexes

A DTR involves four main structures: tendon, muscle, sensory, and motor nerve fibers. When lower extremity neural function is being tested, the examiner taps either the patellar tendon (also called ligament) or the Achilles tendon. The reflex normally elicited by tapping the patellar tendon is the knee jerk and the reflex elicited at the Achilles tendon is the ankle jerk (Table 1-1).

The tap to the tendon lengthens the muscle belly. This lengthening is detected by the muscle spindle. The 1a sensory fibers innervating the muscle transmit this signal proximally along the peripheral nerve. For the knee jerk, the peripheral nerve innervating the quadriceps muscle is the femoral nerve (L2, 3, 4). The femoral nerve arises from the lumbar plexus. The peripheral nerve innervating the triceps surae is the tibial nerve (S1, 2), which arises from the sacral plexus. Once the signal travels through the appropriate plexus, it then is transmitted sequentially through ventral rami, spinal nerves, and dorsal roots. After traveling through the dorsal root and entering the spinal cord, the 1a fiber synapses on an alpha motor neuron at that spinal cord level. The alpha motor neuron subsequently becomes excited and transmits its motor signal sequentially through the ventral root, spinal nerve, ventral rami, plexus, and finally through the peripheral nerve innervating the muscle. The muscle responds with a contraction, indicating that the sensory and motor fibers innervating that muscle are intact. A diminished DTR may indicate peripheral nervous system dysfunction, while an increased DTR may indicate central nervous system dysfunction. The reports on the reliability and validity of DTRs are variable within the literature.[3,4]

Table 1-2 Lower Extremity Myotomes

Myotomal levels	Osteokinematic movement	Muscles
L1–L3	Hip flexion	Iliopsoas
		Rectus femoris
		Sartorius
L3–L4	Knee extension	Quadriceps
L4	Ankle dorsiflexion	Tibialis anterior
L5	Great toe extension	Extensor hallucis longus
S1–S2	Ankle plantarflexion	Gastrocnemius
		Soleus

Lower Extremity Strength Scan

Lower extremity strength testing also is a screening tool used to assess nervous system function in relation to the low back. Generally, the strength scan performed is organized according to the lower extremity myotomes. A myotome in an adult is represented as a group of muscles whose function is most (but not exclusively) indicative of the function of a given level of the spinal cord and the peripheral neural structures related to that spinal cord segment. Table 1-2 provides a listing of myotomes, muscles, and the osteokinematics used to test each myotome in the lower extremity.

Normal strength in the hip flexors represents intact L1 and L2 myotomes. Knee extension represents the L3 myotome. L4 is represented by ankle dorsiflexion. Great toe extension strength reflects the L5 myotome. The S1 myotome is represented by ankle plantar flexor strength. A strength scan is not intended to replace a thorough manual muscle test. If abnormalities are noted on the scan, specific manual muscle tests are then indicated. By using detailed manual muscle testing, it is possible to further differentiate the level of a potential neural lesion. A complete review of the lower extremity anatomy is beyond the scope of this chapter. See other sources for reviews.[1,5,6]

Sensory Evaluation

Information regarding pain, touch, temperature, and position is typically gathered during the sensory function evaluation. Examiners frequently fail to gather pertinent information about sensory function because of a lack of understanding of the function of "sensory" nerves. Skin, the primary organ being examined during a sensory evaluation, requires motor and sensory innervation. Cutaneous nerves, typically referred to as "sensory" nerves, contain fibers that perform sensory and motor function and innervate the skin. Hence, the commonly used term "sensory" nerve is a misnomer. Unless the motor functions of the cutaneous nerves are considered during an evaluation, valuable information can be overlooked. The motor functions of a cutaneous nerve include innervation to visceral structures, specifically, the visceral motor components of a cutaneous nerve service glands, erector pili, and smooth muscle. Therefore, regulating peripheral temperature and the vascular supply to the cutaneous and subcutaneous tissues are the functions of the visceral component of a cutaneous nerve. Trophic changes of the skin and nailbeds and discoloration of the skin are among the signs noted after the function of the visceral component of a cutaneous nerve is lost.

Peripheral nervous system dysfunction concurrent with LBP is typically radicular in nature, meaning that it is related to the segmental levels. More precisely, the peripheral nerve damage that accompanies LBP is typically a result of damage to a neural structure located proximal to the plexus and therefore is uni-segmental. If this is the case, the sensory changes will follow a dermatomal pattern. A dermatome is an area of skin that is innervated by fibers from a single spinal cord segmental level. In the lower extremities, the cutaneous fibers from a single spinal cord segmental level arrive at the dermatome after being carried distally by different peripheral nerves. See Figure 1A-25 to review the cutaneous innervation pattern in the lower extremity. Only in the thorax, where there is no plexus, is a dermatome innervated by a single nerve from a single spinal cord level. In the extremities, dermatomes are innervated by multiple nerves, all of which carry fibers from a given spinal cord segment.

Although there is some variability in the dermatomal patterns between individuals, a working knowledge of an accepted dermatomal map proves clinically useful. See Figure 1A-26 for a visual representation of the dermatomes of the lower quarter. Within the lumbar region the dermatomes are horizontally oriented with a slight inferolateral tendency. The dermatome located in the lumbar region is located approximately two levels below the vertebrae of the same level. Table 1-3 lists the locations and landmarks included within each lower extremity dermatome.

Classically, sensory changes in the lower extremities have been thought to always indicate dysfunction within the nervous system of the lumbar spine or a more peripheral neural structure within the lower extremity. Clearly, when these sensory changes occur concurrent with lower extremity

Table 1-3 Lower Extremity Dermatomes

Dermatome	Location and landmarks
L1	Proximal, anterior thigh
	• Distal to inguinal ligament
L2	Proximal, anterior thigh
	• Inferior to L1
	• Courses inferomedially in thigh
	• Terminates middle one-third of medial thigh
L3	Anterior thigh, medial knee, and proximal medial leg
	• Greater trochanter
	• Anterior mid-thigh
	• Inferior one-third of medial thigh
	• Medial aspect of the knee
	• Proximal medial leg
L4	Anterolateral distal thigh, medial leg, and foot
	• Anterolateral thigh
	• Patella
	• Medial surface of the tibia
	• Medial malleolus
	• Medial foot
	• Great toe
L5	Superolateral buttock, lateral thigh, anterolateral leg, and foot
	• Superior buttock
	• Lateral thigh
	• Lateral knee
	• Fibular head
	• Anterior leg
	• Anterior ankle
	• Middle of foot (second, third, and fourth rays) along dorsum and plantar aspects
S1	Buttock, posterior thigh, leg, and lateral ankle and foot
	• Midsection of posterior buttock
	• Posterior thigh
	• Lateral popliteal fossa
	• Posterolateral leg
	• Lateral malleolus
	• Dorsal and plantar aspects of lateral foot, including fifth digit

Table 1-3 *Continued*

Dermatome	Location and landmarks
S2	Buttock, posterior thigh, leg, and foot
	• Medial buttock
	• Posteromedial thigh
	• Medial popliteal fossa
	• Posterior leg including the Achilles tendon
	• Plantar aspect of calcaneus
S3–S4	Perianal region

weakness and, even more convincingly, concurrent with changes in DTRs, it is highly likely that the source of the sensory change is nervous system dysfunction. However, Travell and Simons[7] have documented paresthesias as a result of muscular and fascial dysfunctions. It is therefore important to note whether you, the examiner, can alter the sensation with a thorough palpatory examination of the muscular and fascial structures, which may refer altered sensations to the region being examined.

Special Tests of Neurologic Function

The clinician uses a number of special tests to evaluate the nervous system. Many of these special tests have as one of their main components producing or examining the tension within neural structures. The straight leg raise (SLR) test, slump test, and various neural tension tests are examples. The straight leg raise is a test routinely performed on patients with LBP. The lower extremity of a supine patient is raised with the knee extended. If back, buttock, or lower extremity pain is elicited, the hip is flexed with the knee held in a flexed position. If this movement does not reproduce the pain, the result is concluded to be positive.[8] Classically, clinicians concluded that a positive result on the SLR test indicated a disc protrusion. A review of the literature does not support this.[9,10] Rather, a positive SLR result indicates that stress is being applied to abnormally sensitive tissues within the neuromeningeal pathway.[10] The SLR test has been modified by a number of individuals to introduce more tension within the neuromeningeal structures.[11-13] These modifications include the introduction of ankle dorsiflexion, neck flexion, and/or medial rotation of the hip.

Without critiquing the conclusions or specificity of this test, the anatomic features involved in the SLR test will be described here. The structures that are pertinent during the SLR test are the sciatic nerve and the proximal neural structures that contribute to it, the connective tissues of the nervous system, the myofascial structures to which the sciatic nerve is related, and the bony landmarks associated with the sciatic nerve. A review of the composition and course of the sciatic nerve should prove helpful because it defines the three-dimensional relationships of the sciatic nerve and the structures that may have an influence on the tension within or on the sciatic nerve.

Fibers from the lumbosacral trunk, the L4 and L5 contributions to the sacral plexus, and fibers from the S1–S4 ventral rami join together to form the sacral plexus. The lower lumbar and sacral spinal cord levels are located in the region of the T12–L1 vertebrae (Figure 1A-27). Because of the differences in spinal cord and vertebral column lengths, lumbar and sacral nerve roots travel inferiorly within the vertebral canal, as the cauda equina, to exit the vertebral column at the appropriate vertebral level. In the lumbar region, the spinal nerves—the union of the nerve roots—exit the vertebral column inferior to the vertebra of the same level. For example, the L5 spinal nerve exits the intervertebral foramen formed by the L5 and S1 vertebrae, inferior to the L5 vertebra (Figure 1A-28). The arrangement for the sacral spinal nerves is different because the sacrum is fused and houses the sacral spinal nerves. The ventral sacral foramina provide exits for the sacral ventral rami. The L4–S3 ventral rami network along the posterior wall of the pelvis to form the sacral plexus. The dorsal sacral foramina provide exits for the sacral dorsal rami, which innervate true back muscles and the dorsal sacral cutaneous regions.

The sciatic nerve is the largest nerve from the sacral plexus and exits the pelvis by traveling through the greater sciatic foramen (Figure 1A-29). This space is bordered by the greater sciatic notch along the posterior aspects of the ilium and ischium, and the sacrospinous ligament. Typically, the sciatic nerve then courses deep to the piriformis muscle (Figure 1A-30), although some variations in this arrangement have been reported.[14,15] Variations include the sciatic nerve coursing superficial to or partially piercing the piriformis muscle. Typically, the sciatic nerve courses inferiorly in the deep buttock, deep to the piriformis and superficial to the gemellus, obturator, and quadratus femoris muscles and enters the posterior thigh lateral to the ischial tuberosity, which is the attachment site for the hamstring muscles. The sciatic nerve travels in the midline of the posterior compartment of the thigh and deep to the long head of the biceps femoris in the mid-thigh. Within the popliteal fossa the sciatic nerve divides into the tibial and common peroneal nerves.

The tibial nerve passes between the two heads of the gastrocnemius and the tibial and fibular heads of the soleus to enter the deep posterior compartment of the leg (Figure 1A-31). The tibial nerve travels distally within the posterior compartment of the leg immediately anterior to the deep transverse crural fascia (Figure 1A-32). At the ankle the tibial nerve courses posterior to the medial malleolus (Figure 1A-33). As the tibial nerve enters the foot, it bifurcates into the medial and lateral plantar nerves. These nerves are located deep to the plantar fascia of the foot and between the first and second layers of the intrinsic foot muscles. The common peroneal nerve exits the popliteal fossa laterally to travel around the fibular neck (Figure 1A-34). In this region the common peroneal nerve bifurcates into the deep and superficial peroneal nerves coursing into the anterior and lateral compartments of the leg, respectively. After innervating the peroneal muscles, the superficial peroneal nerve becomes cutaneous, piercing the deep fascia of the anterolateral leg in its distal one-third and innervates the dorsum of the foot. The deep peroneal nerve, traveling deep within the anterior compartment of the leg, innervates the pre-tibial muscles and eventually becomes cutaneous in the foot. The deep peroneal nerve innervates the skin between the first and second digits on the dorsum of the foot.

The bony landmarks that act as fulcrums for the sciatic nerve are the intervertebral foramina of the L4–L5 and L5–S1 motion segments, the ventral sacral foramina, the greater sciatic foramen, the ischial tuberosity, the popliteal fossa, the fibular neck, and the medial malleolus. Palpable bony landmarks provide attachment for the deep fascia. Therefore, fascia in the regions of palpable bony landmarks may also act to anchor the nerve, creating neural tension. In addition, the nerve branches that become cutaneous provide an additional anchoring location for the nerve that may generate neural tension as they pierce the deep fascia to innervate cutaneous tissues.

Tension within the piriformis, the long head of the biceps femoris, the gastrocnemius, the soleus, and the first and second layers of the intrinsic foot muscles may also generate neural tension as the sciatic nerve and its branches course deep to these muscles. In some cases the sciatic nerve may actually pierce the piriformis, thereby potentially creating greater amounts of neural tension. Morphologic or physiologic shortening of the muscles noted above may contribute to this tension in the neural structures. During the SLR test and neural tension tests in general, each of these muscles is put on stretch to determine the effect on the sciatic nerve.

The connective tissue elements of the nervous system may also increase neural tension. The spinal cord is surrounded by three layers of connective tissues: the superficial dura mater, the arachnoid mater, and the deep pia mater. The dura mater is anchored at its superior aspect as it surrounds the brain, enclosed within the cranium, and is anchored at its inferior aspect to the anterior aspect of the sacral canal at the S2 level. Any posturing or movement that increases the distance between the inferior and superior aspects of the dura mater will create tension within this structure. Therefore, a loss in the normal spinal curvatures will place tension on the dura mater and the structures it surrounds. The flexion created as the patient flexes the head and neck during the SLR test or during the slump test increases the distances between the "attachments" of the dura mater. The dura mater continues into the peripheral nervous system as the epineurium, which is the outermost layer of connective tissue surrounding peripheral nerves. Thus, tension may be transmitted from the peripheral structures to those central or conversely, from the central structures to the peripheral structures.

As highlighted in the previous discussion, the interconnections of tissues facilitate tension generation. The fact that forces are transmitted between interconnected tissues gives rise to the potential for the generation of tension. Making these relationships even more complex is the fact that each of these structures (bones, muscles, fascia, connective tissues of the nervous system) is innervated. Therefore, each of these structures may also be sources of pain or of pain referral in and of themselves, regardless of their ability to produce tension within the neural structures. Again we are left with the question, "What is the source of the symptoms and signs produced by an SLR or 'neural' tension test?"

Anatomic Features of Space-Occupying Lesions

Effective evaluation and treatment of a patient with LBP are augmented when the examiner is able to identify the structures that have the potential to compress the nerve roots or spinal nerves. The structures most frequently involved in lumbar space-occupying lesions of the nervous system are those structures related to the intervertebral foramina.

The intervertebral foramen is bordered superiorly and inferiorly by the pedicles of adjacent vertebrae (Figure 1A-35). These portions of the pedicle are named the inferior and superior vertebral notches, respectively. The anterior wall of the intervertebral foramen is formed by the posterolateral aspects of the vertebral bodies and the adjoining disc. The posterior wall of the intervertebral foramen is formed by the anterior portion of the ipsilateral facet joint. Specifically, the structures located in this region are the anterior capsule of the facet joint reinforced by the ligamentum flavum. Spinal stenosis is the diagnosis indicating narrowing of the intervertebral foramen. Any positional fault of the vertebrae closing down the intervertebral foramen or encroachment of the space by some structure not normally found here may lead to a lesion of the spinal nerve within the intervertebral foramen. Objects most frequently encroaching in this space are displaced discs, facet joint osteophytes, or an abnormal thickening of the ligamentum flavum. Loss of disc height, as experienced in the aging process, may also limit the size of the intervertebral foramen.

Anatomic Features on Palpation

Much can be learned by placing one's hands on the patient during examination. Information concerning the condition of the tissues being palpated, such as temperature, turgor, and tenderness, can be gained. Position and mobility information from the structures can also be gained. Before determining if the structures being palpated are normal, it is imperative that the examiner appreciate exactly what structures are being palpated. Additionally, because of the frequent use of computed tomographic (CT) and magnetic resonance imaging (MRI) scans, the ability to understand three-dimensional relationships of the low back is important. The anatomic features palpable in the low back will be described in the following paragraphs according to depth, progressing from medial to lateral, posteriorly then anteriorly.

Thoracolumbar Fascia

Beginning most superficially in the low back, the examiner contacts the skin, subcutaneous fat, and superficial fascia. All of these structures are innervated and thus must be considered as possible sources of pain. Progressing deeper, the examiner contacts the thoracolumbar fascia. This is a thick layer of fascia with several layers separating the various groups of muscles in the low back. The deep fascia, because it is a noncontractile tissue largely composed of relatively unorganized fibers, provides a firmer resistance to the examiner's hands.

It is important to understand the compartmentalization provided by the layers of the thoracolumbar fascia (Figure 1A-36). The interconnections of the fascia of the posterior abdominal wall, the erector spinae, and the transversospinalis muscle groups may lead to shared dysfunction. For example, fascial restrictions surrounding the psoas major may lead to increased tension within the fascia of the quadratus lumborum and consequently the erector spinae.

The deep layer of the thoracolumbar fascia is trilaminar in the lumbar region. The posterior layer attaches medially to the lumbar spinous processes, the median sacral crest, and the lumbar supraspinous ligaments. An unnamed layer of fascia progresses anteriorly from the posterior layer to separate the multifidus from the erector spinae. This unnamed layer attaches to the medial portion of the transverse processes. The middle layer of the thoracolumbar fascia attaches to the tips of the lumbar transverse processes and adjoining intertransverse ligaments. Superiorly, this middle layer attaches to the inferior aspect of the twelfth rib and inferiorly to the iliac crest. This middle layer separates the anterior fibers of the erector spinae from the quadratus lumborum. The anterior layer of the thoracolumbar fascia covers the anterior aspect of the quadratus lumborum and medially attaches to the anterior aspects of the lumbar transverse processes. The deep fascia surrounding the psoas major unites with the anterior layer of the thoracolumbar fascia anterior to the lumbar transverse processes. The posterior and middle layers of the thoracolumbar fascia unite at the lateral margin of the erector spinae, specifically the iliocostalis, to form the aponeurotic posterior attachment of the abdominal muscles.

Palpating Posterior Muscles of the Low Back

Beginning most medially in the lumbar region, the muscle mass immediately off the midline is the multifidus, which is the middle layer of the transversospinalis muscle group (see Figures 1A-6, 1A-8). This is the largest true back muscle in the lumbar region and is the only muscle of the transversospinalis group that is significantly developed in the lumbar region. The multifidus is composed of multiple laminae, the more superficial fibers crossing five motion segments. In general, the multifidus attaches the mamillary process of the articular pillar to the lamina of the vertebrae two to five segments superiorly. The fiber direction of the multifidus is superomedial, but is difficult to detect on palpation because of the aponeurosis covering the multifidus. Increased turgor noted within the muscle may make the detection of fiber direction clearer. The most inferior fibers of the multifidus attach to the dorsal surface of the sacrum and posterior inferior iliac spine.

Thus, when palpating the dorsal surface of the sacrum and the posterior inferior iliac spine, the examiner is palpating through the aponeurosis of the erector spinae and into the fibers of the multifidus. Some refer to this region as the sacral sulcus. The width of the multifidus is such that it generally fills in the space between the articular pillars and the medial portions of the lamina throughout the lumbar region. This space generally measures 2–3 cm. Given that this is not a great distance and yet the multifidus muscle holds the claim as the largest of the lumbar muscles, it is correct to conclude that the multifidus has considerable depth.

The muscles of the posterior thigh and the hamstrings all share proximal attachment to the ischial tuberosity, which is easily palpable along the medial aspect of the gluteal fold. The medial hamstrings—the semimembranosus and semitendinosus—and the lateral hamstring—the biceps femoris long head—become more easily distinguishable from one another distally in the thigh. The tendon of the biceps femoris can be palpated at the knee posterior to the iliotibial band and also as it attaches to the fibular head. Coursing in the posterior thigh, the semitendinosus is located medial to the semimembranosus. This relationship changes at the knee, as the semitendinosus attaches more anteromedially.

The rectus femoris and the sartorius are palpable anterior thigh muscles that cross the hip and attach to the pelvis. The straplike sartorius, which attaches to the anterior superior iliac spine (ASIS), is the more superficial of these muscles and descends toward the medial leg. The sartorius forms the lateral border of the femoral triangle (Figure 1A-37). The rectus femoris, which also is palpable as it attaches to the anterior inferior iliac spine (AIIS) and the rim of the acetabulum, courses longitudinally along the anterior thigh and joins the quadriceps tendon at the knee.

All medial compartment muscles attach to the pelvis and may affect the lumbar spine. The pectineus, which forms the medial floor of the femoral triangle (see Figure 1A-37), is the most anterior of the adductor muscles (see Figure 1A-18). Medial to the pectineus, forming the medial border of the femoral triangle, is the adductor longus. The adductor longus can be palpated as it descends laterally toward the middle one-third of the femoral shaft. The adductor brevis is not directly palpable, being located deep to the superior portion of the adductor longus. Forming the most posterior portion of the medial thigh compartment is the adductor magnus. This muscle mass is most easily distinguishable by first locating the medial hamstrings. The muscle mass immediately anterior to the medial hamstrings is the adductor magnus. The straplike gracilis is the medial-most muscle descending the medial compartment of the thigh, and although it is difficult to identify, it is most palpable in the mid-section of the thigh.

Anatomic Features During Palpation for Position

The examiner's goal in palpating for position is to determine if a positional fault is present. Where is the bone in relation to the other osseous structures? To distinguish a positional fault, one must understand normal vertebral positions and the relationships of the bony elements to one another. The normal alignment of the bony elements of the spine are reviewed here and the more common positional faults are described.

Normal Alignment

The bony elements palpable from the dorsal aspect of the spine include the spinous processes, the articular pillars, and the transverse processes (Figure 1A-38). In the thoracic spine the transversocostal joints can also be palpated. In the lumbar region the spinous processes are large, hatchet-shaped structures directed posteriorly. In the thoracic spine the spinous processes are long and inferiorly directed. The thoracic spinous processes overlap the spinous processes of the vertebra inferior to them (Figure 1A-39). Specifically, the tip of a typical middle or lower thoracic spinous process extends one to two finger breadths inferior to that vertebral level. If the vertebra is in the normal sagittal plane position (i.e., neither flexed or extended beyond the normal position), the distance between adjacent spinous processes will be equivalent (Figure 1A-40).

The transverse processes of the vertebrae are also different between the regions of the spine (Figure 1A-41). The thoracic transverse processes point laterally, posteriorly, and superiorly and have a rather bulbous end, which articulates with the rib. In the lumbar region, the transverse processes point laterally and are slender compared with those of the thoracic region. The thoracic transverse processes are directly palpable, especially laterally as they form the transversocostal joints, articulating with the tubercles of the ribs. The lumbar transverse processes are not usually directly palpable because of the large muscle mass overlying them, but can be perceived indirectly. If the vertebrae are in a normal transverse plane position (i.e., no rotational deformity), the transverse processes will be an equal distance from the dorsal surface (see Figure 1A-36). This relationship assumes equality of soft-tissue depth bilaterally. Normal transverse plane position can also be evaluated by examining the position of the spinous processes in relation to the midline. Normal transverse plane position is indicated if the spinous processes are vertically aligned with one another in the midline (Figure 1A-42A).

Positional Faults of Vertebrae

It must be kept in mind that the reliability of spinal positional data is in question. A thorough review of that literature is beyond the scope of this chapter. Even if palpation of vertebral position is reliable, conclusions drawn from positional faults must be viewed with caution in light of the potential for bony variations. For example, a bony variation may lead one to conclude that a vertebra is rotated when in fact the spinous process is simply deviated laterally. The question also exists about the relationship between position and function. If a vertebra is found to be "out," can it be assumed that this segment is a source of pain or dysfunction? In light of this, palpation for mobility is the more crucial of the palpatory tests.

A flexed or extended vertebra would represent a positional fault in the sagittal plane. Normal sagittal plane alignment is indicated by similar distances between adjacent spinous processes (see Figure 1A-40). Generally, spinal flexion increases the distance between successive spinous processes (Figure 1A-43) and extension decreases this distance (Figure 1A-44). If it is noted that the distance between adjacent spinous processes is asymmetric, one must determine which vertebra is out of position and in which direction the vertebra has moved.

Figure 1A-45 gives examples of sagittal plane motion segment positional faults. Flexion of a vertebra would move that spinous process more superiorly, thus diminishing the distance to the spinous process superior to it. Likewise, flexion would also move the spinous process of that vertebra farther away from the spinous process of the vertebra inferior to it. In short, flexion of a vertebra decreases the space superior to its spinous process and increases the space inferior to its spinous process. Extension of a vertebra increases the space superior to its spinous process and decreases the space inferior to its spinous process.

A rotated vertebra would indicate a positional fault in the transverse plane. Normal transverse plane alignment is indicated when the transverse processes are equivalent distances from the dorsal aspect of the trunk, again assuming symmetry of soft tissues lateral to the spine. Thus, if it is noted that one transverse process appears more posteriorly located relative to the contralateral transverse process, a transverse plane positional fault may be indicated. The examiner must then determine which vertebra has moved and in which direction the vertebra has rotated. Posterior movement of the right transverse process is accompanied by movement of the left transverse process of the same vertebra in the anterior direction. Rotation of the spine is named in relation to a motion segment, not a vertebra. The positional fault is named according to the superior vertebra of the motion segment. For example, if the L2 right transverse process is noted to be in a posterior position and the L1 and L3 vertebrae are in normal positions, the positional fault is named according to the L2–L3 motion segment. Specifically, the L2–L3 motion segment is in a position of right rotation (see Figure 1A-42B, C).

A rotated motion segment can also be detected if the spinous process is deviated from the midline. For example, during right rotation the spinous process deviates to the left. Thus, if the spinous process of L2 is positioned to the left of midline and the L1 and L3 spinous processes are located in the midline, the motion segment of L2–L3 is in a position of right rotation (Figure 1A-46).

The examiner must be careful not to treat an apparent positional fault that may simply be a variation from the normal osseous structure. The mobility of the segment must be the benchmark that indicates the need for mobilization of that particular motion segment. For example, despite the fact that the L2–L3 motion segment appears to be rotated to the right, does the motion segment rotate normally in both directions? To answer this question, the examiner must palpate for mobility.

Anatomic Features During Palpation for Mobility

Joints of the Vertebral Column

Before determining if normal motion exists at a particular motion segment, the examiner must understand the joint and the structures that limit motion at that joint. The typical motion segment in the lumbar spine is composed of three joints, the joint between the anterior elements of adjacent vertebrae and the paired joints between the posterior elements of adjacent vertebrae. The anterior element of a vertebra is made of up the vertebral bodies. The posterior element of a vertebra is composed of the pedicles, transverse processes, lamina, superior and inferior articular processes, and the spinous process.

Specifically, adjacent vertebral bodies articulate via the intervertebral disc to form the intervertebral joint (see Figure 1A-35). The intervertebral joint, more precisely called the anterior intervertebral joint, is a symphyseal joint and is by definition a cartilaginous synarthrodial joint. Unlike diarthrodial (synovial) joints, the anterior intervertebral joints have no joint space and the joint surfaces are joined together by a fibrocartilaginous disc. The fibrocartilaginous disc is reinforced by collagenous ligaments (annulus). Although symphysis joints do not permit the degree of motion available at synovial joints, there is appreciable movement present.

The nomenclature of the posterior joints of the low back is not as consistent. The paired joints formed by the articulation of adjacent superior and inferior articular processes are generally referred to as facet joints (Figure 1A-47). More precisely, these joints are referred to as *zygapophyseal joints* or *posterior intervertebral joints*. The facet joints are diarthrodial joints; thus, they possess a joint space, a capsule, a synovial membrane and fluid, and joint surfaces covered by articular cartilage. As discussed earlier in this chapter, the orientation of the facet joints in part determines the osteokinematic and arthrokinematic movements available at that motion segment. The soft tissues supporting each of these joints and connecting the vertebrae are other factors that determine the motions available at facet joints.

Ligaments of the Low Back

The tissues adjoining the vertebral bodies are the anterior and posterior longitudinal ligaments and the intervertebral disc (Figures 1A-48, 1A-49, 1A-50). The longitudinal ligaments attach to the anterior and posterior aspects of the vertebral bodies and adjoining discs throughout the spine. The tissues adjoining the posterior elements are the ligamentum flavum—which is a ligament with greater amounts of elastin attaching adjacent lamina—and the interspinous and intertransverse ligaments attaching adjacent spinous and transverse processes, respectively. Also present are intrinsic ligaments (thickenings of the facet joint capsules), which adjoin the adjacent articular pillars. The lumbosacral ligaments attach the lower lumbar vertebrae to the sacrum (Figure 1A-51). The posterior and anterior sacroiliac ligaments cross the sacroiliac joint and assist in stabilizing the sacrum on the innominate bone. Finally, the sacrotuberous and the sacrospinous ligaments attach the sacrum to the ischium and in so doing complete the lesser and greater sciatic foramina, respectively (Figure 1A-52).

All ligaments of the spine are innervated, as is the capsule of the facet joint, and may be sources of pain. Similarly, the most external portion of the annulus fibrosus is innervated. Specifically, the facet joints and the ligaments of the posterior element are innervated by the medial, intermediate, and lateral branches of the lumbar dorsal rami. Surrounding the vertebral body is a large plexus of nerve fibers formed from the lumbar sympathetic trunks and branches of the ventral rami. It is from this plexus, in addition to the sinuvertebral nerve (a retrograde branch from the ventral rami) and gray rami communicans, that the vertebrae, longitudinal ligaments, and periphery of the annulus fibrosus receive innervation.

In general, the function of posteriorly located structures is to limit spinal flexion. Conversely, the anterior spinal structures limit spinal extension. The amount of forward flexion normally exceeds that of extension; thus, there are more posterior ligaments than anterior ligaments. There are also osseous structures that limit extension, thus minimizing the need for anterior ligaments.

Arthrokinematics of Motion Segments

An understanding of spinal arthrokinematics will assist the examiner in determining which of the soft tissues may be limiting osteokinematic functions. During open chain flexion of the lumbar spine, which is indicated by the superior vertebra moving, the superior vertebra of the motion segment slides in the superior direction, or "upslides." During open chain extension of the lumbar spine, the superior vertebra of the motion segment slides in the inferior direction, or "downslides." Because of the facet orientation in the lumbar spine, anterior motion of the vertebra is limited. The superior lumbar segments are more limited in anterior slide than the inferior lumbar segments because of the J shape of their facets. Although not as dramatic as noted in the cervical spine, the superior vertebra of the motion segment slides anteriorly with open chain flexion and posteriorly with open chain extension.

During rotation of the lumbar spine, the articular processes move in the transverse plane. The ipsilateral facet joint "gaps" with rotation of the lumbar spine (Figure 1A-53). The joint surfaces move away from one another. In other words, the capsule of the ipsilateral facet joint undergoes tensile force and becomes taut. The transverse process of the ipsilateral side moves posteriorly, indicating that the ipsilateral posterior elements are moving posteriorly. In comparison, the contralateral facet joint undergoes compressive forces, causing the contralateral facet joint capsule to become slack.

The osteokinematic motions of sidebending or lateral flexion occur in the frontal plane. The facet joint on the ipsilateral side undergoes compressive force during sidebending. In other words, the facet joint surfaces approximate one another. The contralateral facet joint "gaps" during sidebending. More precisely, the contralateral articular processes move away from each other during lateral flexion, thereby creating a tensile force. Thus, the contralateral facet joint capsule becomes taut, while the ipsilateral side becomes slack.

The relationships noted above during cardinal plane movement obviously change as one considers that most movements do not occur purely in cardinal planes. For example, the compression and tensile forces generated in the facet joints during lumbar rotation are altered when the spine is concurrently flexed or extended. Making these relationships even more complex is the fact that spinal motions are inextricably coupled. In other words, the spine cannot move in a pure transverse or frontal plane, even when desired. Lovett[14] was the first to record the coupling of lumbar motions, which became apparent during his study of scoliosis. In the years that followed, numerous authors[15–24] reported various coupling patterns throughout the spine, at times in conflict with one another. Much of the controversy centers on the changes in the coupling pattern between rotation and sidebending noted when the spine is positioned in various degrees of flexion or extension.

Figure 1A-54 presents a summary of the spinal regional coupling patterns as they are now accepted. It is generally accepted that lumbar lateral flexion and contralateral rotation are coupled within a neutral sagittal plane spine. The lumbar spinous processes move in the same direction as the sidebending. Thus, the segment rotates away from the sidebending when the lumbar spine is in its normal lordotic posture. When the spine is in a flexed posture, the rotation of the lumbar vertebra is toward the sidebending. Pearcy et al.,[23] noted a difference at the lumbosacral motion segment. These researchers found that the L5–S1 motion segment couples motions like the cervical spine—that is, L5–S1 rotate toward the sidebending (Figure 1A-55).

Coupling of vertebral motions has functional anatomic significance in that, during lateral flexion, the structures that are limiting rotation will also be stressed. Given that spinal rotation places the greatest stress on the annulus fibrosus and is not uncommonly a mechanism of injury to the low back, it is prudent to keep in mind the coupling relationships as you examine and treat patients with LBP. One could hypothesize that the increased motion and incidence of pathologic conditions at the L4–L5 segment may be related to the transition in lumbar coupling relationships.

Soft Tissues Restricting Vertebral Motion

Generally, structures located posteriorly on the vertebrae become taut during spinal flexion because of the "upslide" and anterior motion of the vertebrae. Thus, during flexion, the posterior longitudinal, interspinous, and intertransverse ligaments undergo tension. The posterior portion of the annulus as well as the ligamentum flavum also experience tension. As a general rule, the more posterior the soft-tissue structure is located, the more elongation is required of that structure during spinal flexion. Bilateral facet joint capsules also undergo tension during flexion.

During spinal extension, the posterior soft tissues undergo shortening concurrent with the compressive forces generated at the facet joints. The anterior longitudinal ligament and the anterior portion of the annulus experience tension during spinal extension. Posterior-anterior (PA) glides thus stress the same tissues.

Rotation of the spine creates greatest tension in the annular fibers, and for this reason, rotation is the osteokinematic movement that maximally stresses the annulus. It is hypothesized that all other osteokinematic movements cause less than 50% of the annulus to undergo tension because of the oblique and alternating fiber orientation of the concentric annular rings (Figure 1A-56). Because none of the ligaments of the spine have a purely horizontal fiber direction, none of the spinal ligaments become maximally taut during rotation. Spinal rotation does, however, have a significant effect on the facet joint capsules and ligaments. During rotation, the ipsilateral facet joint capsule is put on stretch and undergoes tension. Rotational glides thus stress the same tissues.

During lateral flexion of the spine, the contralateral facet joint capsule and ligaments undergo tension. Likewise, all structures on the contralateral side undergo tension during lateral flexion. Specifically, the contralateral intertransverse ligament, the ligamentum flavum, and a portion of the laterally located annular fibers undergo tension. Although the degree of tension is diminished, it is biomechanically possible that the contralateral half of the anterior and posterior longitudinal ligaments undergo tension during lateral flexion as well.

References

1. Williams PL, Bannister LH, Berry MM, et al. Gray's Anatomy (38th ed) New York: Churchill Livingstone, 1995;812.
2. White AA, Panjabi MM. Clinical Biomechanics of the Spine (2nd ed). Philadelphia: Lippincott, 1990;106.
3. Basmajian JV, Nyberg R. Rational Manual Therapies. Baltimore: Williams & Wilkins, 1993;135.
4. Yates DA. Unilateral lumbo-sacral nerve compression. Ann Phys Med 1964;7:169.
5. Moore KL. Clinically Oriented Anatomy (3rd ed). Baltimore: Williams & Wilkins, 1992.
6. Jenkins DB. Hollinshead's Functional Anatomy of the Limbs and Back (6th ed). Philadelphia: Saunders, 1991.
7. Travell JG, Simons DG. Myofascial Pain and Dysfunction: The Trigger Point Manual. Baltimore: Williams & Wilkins, 1992.
8. Urban LM. The straight-leg raising test: a review. J Orthop Sports Phys Ther 1981;2:117.
9. Grieve GP. Sciatica and the straight-leg-raising test in manipulative treatment. Physiotherapy 1970;56:337.
10. Brody IA, Wilkins RJ. The signs of Kernig and Brudzinski. Neurological classics XXI. Arch Neurol 1969;21:215.
11. Brudzinski J. A new sign of the lower extremities in meningitis of children (neck sign). Neurological classics XXI. Arch Neurol 1969;21:217.
12. Wartenberg R. The signs of Brudzinski and of Kernig. J Pediatr 1950;37:679.
13. Lee CS, Tsai TL. The relationship of the sciatic nerve to the piriformis muscle. J Formosam Med Assoc 1974;73:75–80.
14. Lovett RW. The mechanism of the normal spine in relation to scoliosis. Med Surg J 1905;153:349.
15. Lysell E. Motion in the cervical spine. Acta Orthop Scand 1969;Suppl 123:1.
16. Miles M, Sullivan WE. Lateral bending at the lumbar and lumbosacral joints. Anat Rec 1961;139:387.

17. Moroney SP, Schultz AB, Miller JAA, Andersson GBJ. Load-displacement properties of lower cervical spine motion segments. J Biomech 1988;21:769.
18. Panjabi MM, Brand RA, White AA. Three dimensional flexibility and stiffness properties of the human thoracic spine. J Biomech 1976;9:185.
19. Panjabi MM, Krag M, White AA, Southwick WO. Effects of preload on load-displacement curves of the lumbar spine. Orthop Clin North Am 1977;8:181.
20. Panjabi MM, Summers DJ, Pelker RR, et al. Three-dimensional load displacement curves of the cervical spine. J Orthop Res 1986;4:152.
21. Panjabi MM, Yamamoto I, Oxland T, Crisco JJ. How does posture affect the coupling? Spine 1989;14:1002.
22. Pearcy M, Portek I, Shepherd J. Three-dimensional X-ray analysis of normal movement in the lumbar spine. Spine 1984;9:294.
23. Pearcy MJ, Tibrewal SB. Axial rotation and lateral bending in the normal lumbar spine measured by three-dimensional radiography. Spine 1984;9:582.
24. Pearcy MJ. Stereo radiography of lumbar spine motion. Acta Orthop Scand Suppl 1985;212:1.

Chapter 1
Appendixes

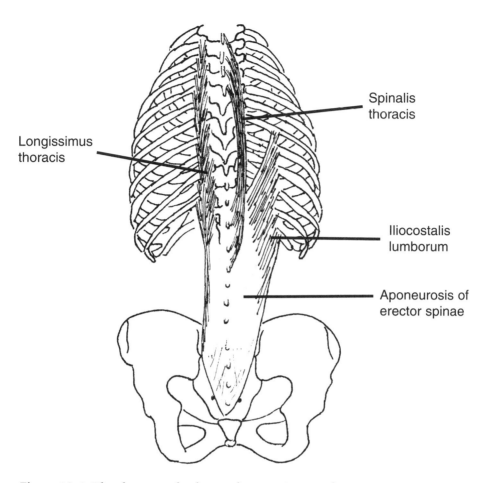

Figure 1A-4 The three true back muscles constituting the erector spinae group, which influences the low back.

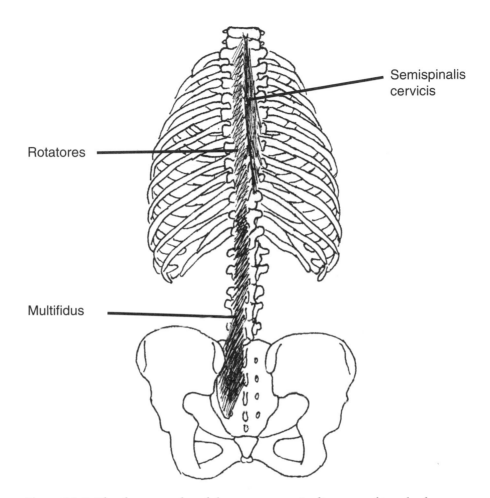

Semispinalis
cervicis

Rotatores

Multifidus

Figure 1A-5 The three muscles of the transversospinalis group of true back muscles. Note that the development of the multifidus is greatest in the lumbar region, the rotatores in the thoracic region, and the semispinalis in the cervical region.

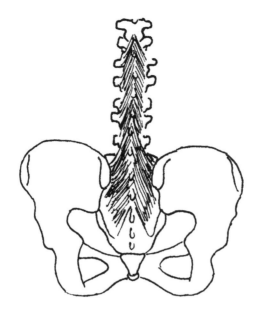

Figure 1A-6 Multifidus. Note the superomedial direction of the fibers.

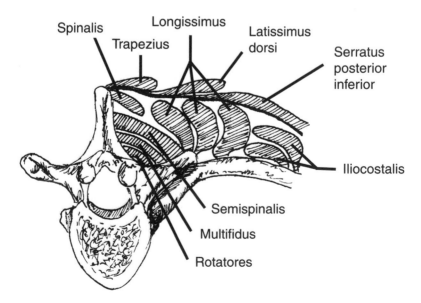

Figure 1A-7 Transverse section through the thoracic region displaying the depth relationships of the muscles.

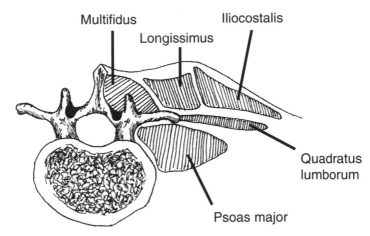

Figure 1A-8 Transverse section through the lumbar region displaying the depth relationships of the muscles.

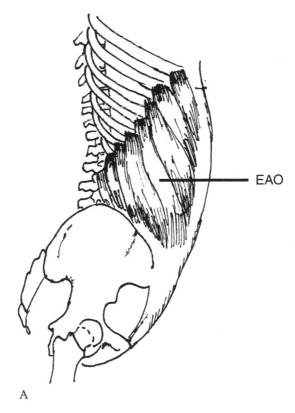

Figure 1A-9 The abdominal muscles. (A) Lateral view of the trunk. (EAO = external abdominal oblique.)

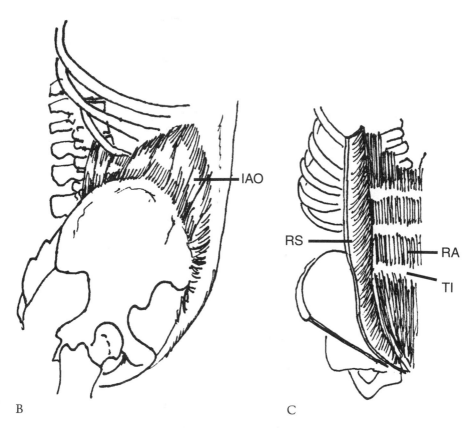

B   C

Figure 1A-9 *Continued* (B) Lateral view of the trunk. (C) Anterior view of the trunk. (IAO = internal abdominal oblique; RA = rectus abdominus; RS = rectus sheath; TI = tendinous inscriptions.)

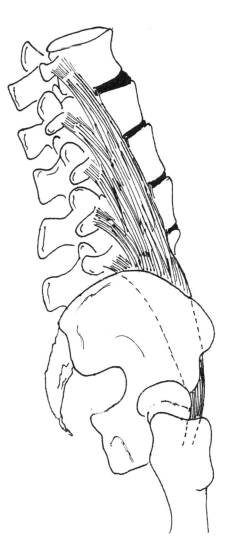

Figure 1A-10 Lateral view of the psoas major.

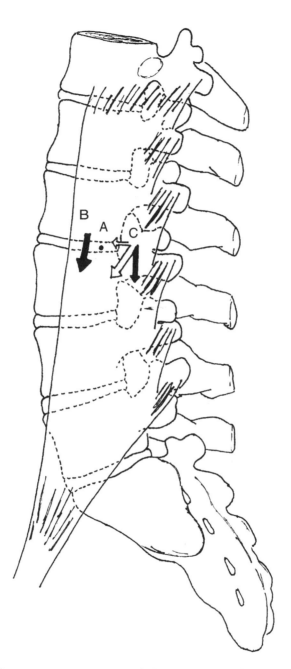

Figure 1A-11 Schematic representation of the psoas major. (A = axis of rotation; B = fibers of the psoas major coursing anterior to the axis and hence capable of flexing the spine; C = fibers of the psoas major coursing posterior to the axis and hence capable of extending the spine.)

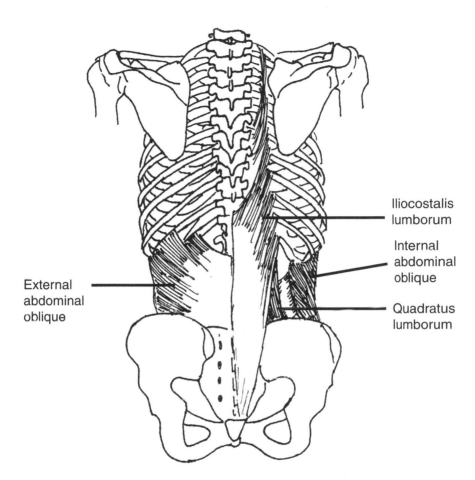

Iliocostalis
lumborum

Internal
abdominal
oblique

External
abdominal
oblique

Quadratus
lumborum

Figure 1A-12 Lateral flexors of the low back.

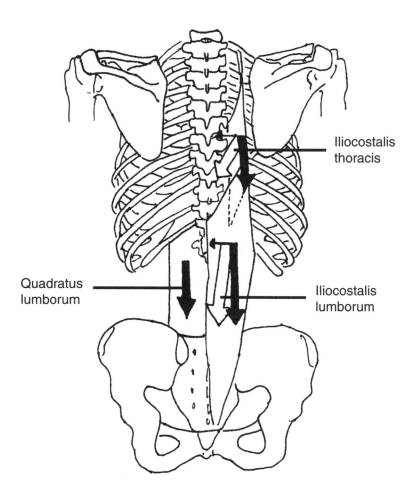

Figure 1A-13 Schematic representation of the fiber direction of the lateral flexors of the spine. Note that the iliocostalis lumborum and iliocostalis thoracis have larger longitudinal components than rotational components and hence are more efficient lateral flexors than rotators of the spine.

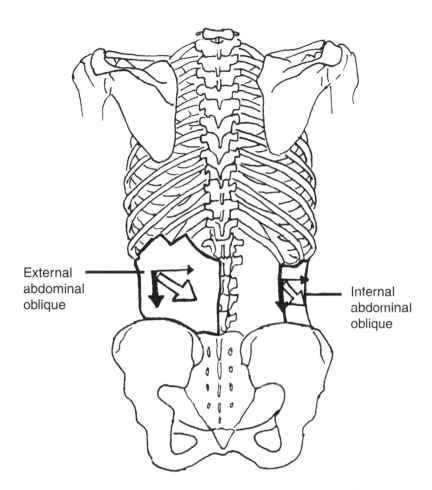

Figure 1A-14 The transverse and longitudinal components of the abdominal muscles producing trunk rotation and lateral flexion, respectively.

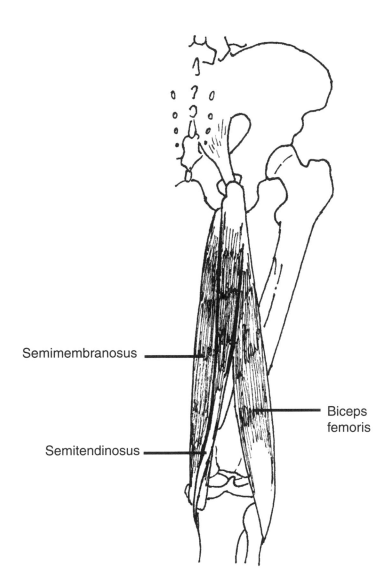

Figure 1A-17 Muscles of the posterior thigh compartment attaching to the innominate bone.

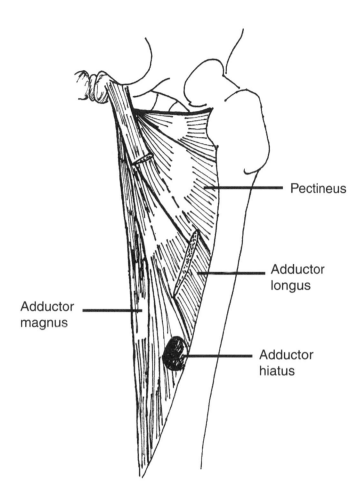

Figure 1A-18 Muscles of the medial thigh compartment attaching to the innominate bone.

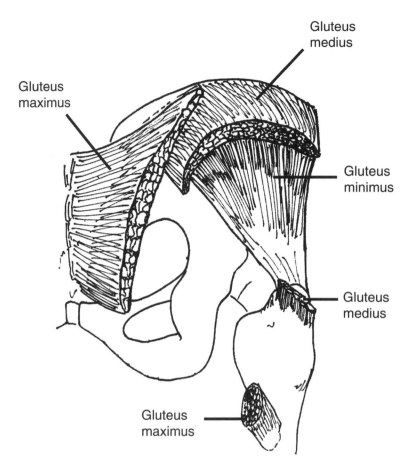

Figure 1A-19 Muscles of the buttock attaching to the pelvis.

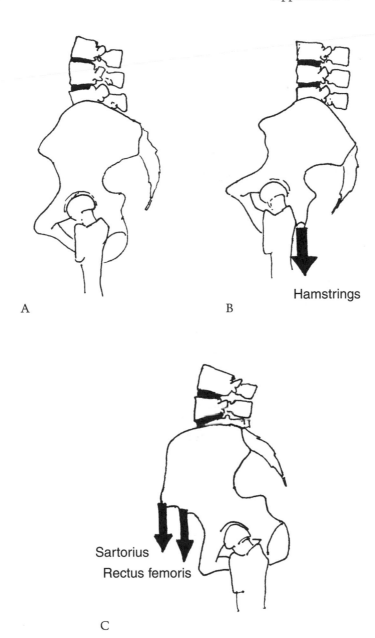

Figure 1A-20 Sagittal plane pelvic positions. (A) Normal alignment. (B) Posterior pelvic tilt. (C) Anterior pelvic tilt.

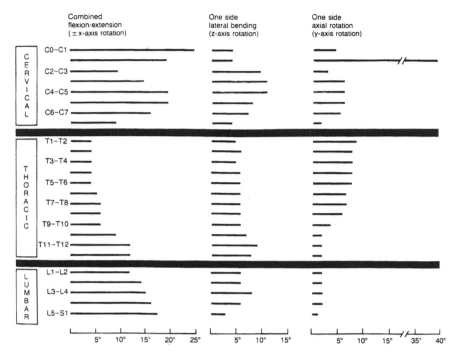

Figure 1A-21 The motion available in cardinal planes at each spinal motion segment. (Reprinted with permission from AA White, MM Panjabi. Clinical Biomechanics of the Spine [2nd ed]. Philadelphia: Lippincott, 1990;106.) This is an updated composite of what the authors consider, based on careful review of the literature, to be the most representative values for rotatory ranges of motion at different levels of the spine (in the traditional planes of motion).

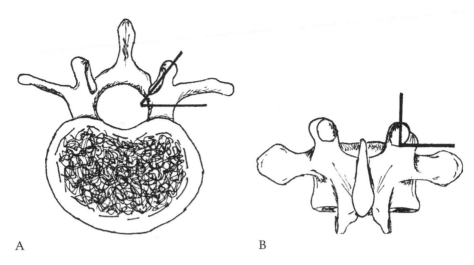

A   B

Figure 1A-22 Typical orientation of the lumbar facets. (A) Forty-five degrees from the frontal plane. (B) Ninety degrees from the transverse plane.

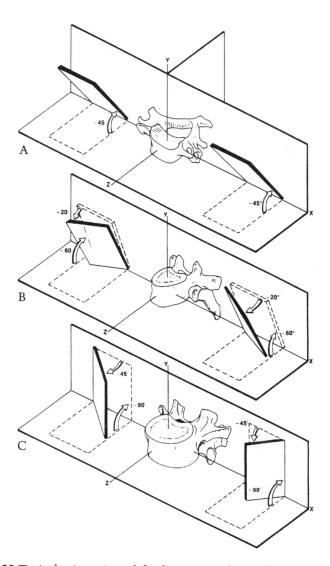

Figure 1A-23 Typical orientation of the facets in each spinal region. A graphical representation of the facet joint inclinations in various regions of the spine is obtained by rotating two cards lying in the horizontal plane through two consecutive angles, x-axis rotation followed by y-axis rotation. Typical values for the two angles for the three regions of the spine are (A) cervical spine: –45 degrees followed by 0 degrees; (B) thoracic spine: –60 degrees followed by +20 degrees for the right facet or –20 degrees for the left facet; (C) lumbar spine: –90 degrees and 45 degrees for the right facet or +45 degrees for the left facet. These are only rough estimates. There are variations within the regions of the spine and between individuals. (Reprinted with permission from AA White, MM Panjabi. Clinical Biomechanics of the Spine [2nd ed]. Philadelphia: Lippincott, 1990;30.)

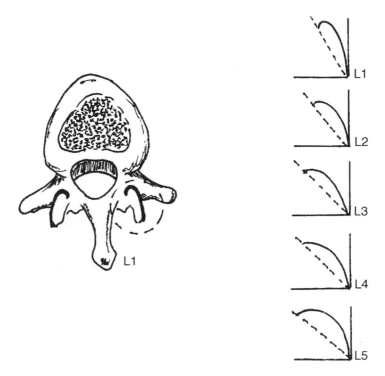

Figure 1A-24 Superior view of L1 vertebra. Note the orientation of the facet to the frontal plane. The schematic demonstrates the J shape of the upper facets and the transition to the more open, C-shaped L5 facets.

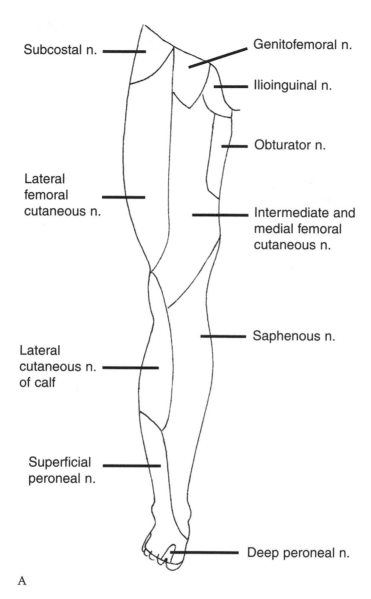

Subcostal n.

Genitofemoral n.

Ilioinguinal n.

Obturator n.

Lateral femoral cutaneous n.

Intermediate and medial femoral cutaneous n.

Saphenous n.

Lateral cutaneous n. of calf

Superficial peroneal n.

Deep peroneal n.

A

Figure 1A-25 Cutaneous innervation of the lower extremity. (A) Anterior view. (B) Posterior view.

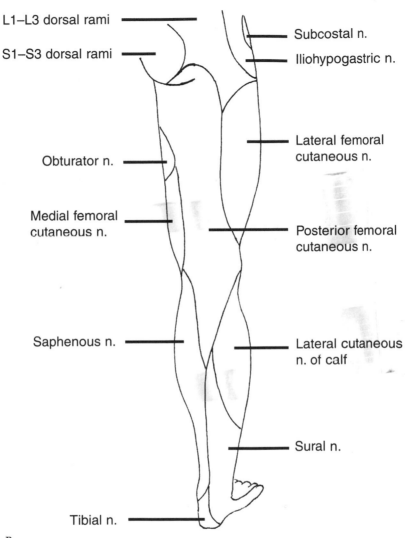

L1–L3 dorsal rami

S1–S3 dorsal rami

Subcostal n.

Iliohypogastric n.

Obturator n.

Lateral femoral cutaneous n.

Medial femoral cutaneous n.

Posterior femoral cutaneous n.

Saphenous n.

Lateral cutaneous n. of calf

Sural n.

Tibial n.

B

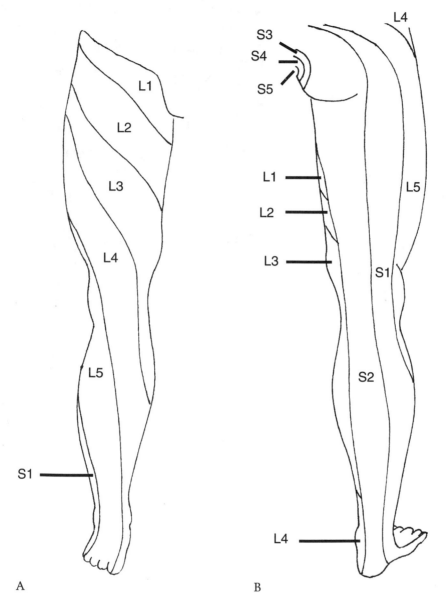

A   B

Figure 1A-26 Dermatomal pattern in the lower extremity. (A) Anterior view. (B) Posterior view.

Spinal cord levels   **Vertebral levels**

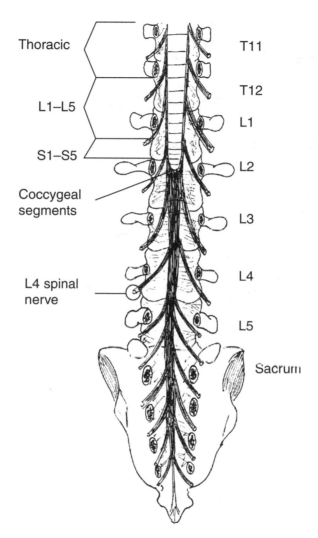

Figure 1A-27 Posterior view of the vertebral column after laminectomies have been performed to expose the vertebral canal. The contents of the vertebral canal, the spinal cord, and the cauda equina are represented at the appropriate levels for an adult. Note the vertebral levels on the right and the spinal cord levels on the upper left. The roots, joining together to form the spinal nerves, are shown exiting through the intervertebral foramen.

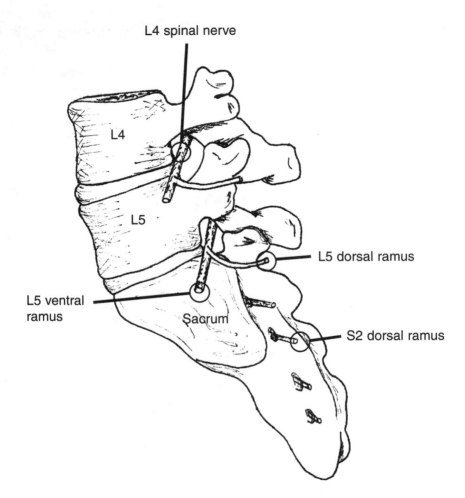

Figure 1A-28 Lateral view of the L4–L5 and L5–S1 motion segments. Note the L4 and L5 spinal nerves exiting the intervertebral foramina and dividing into dorsal and ventral rami. The sacral dorsal rami are exiting the dorsal sacral foramina.

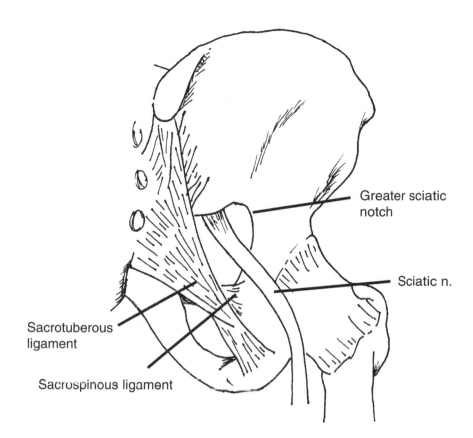

Figure 1A-29 Posterior view of the pelvis and hip demonstrating the course of the sciatic nerve.

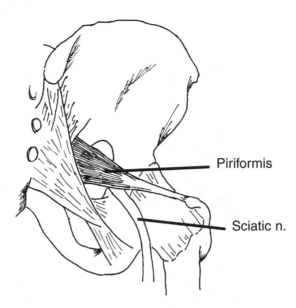

Piriformis

Sciatic n.

Figure 1A-30 Posterior view of the pelvis and hip demonstrating the typical relationship of the sciatic nerve and the piriformis.

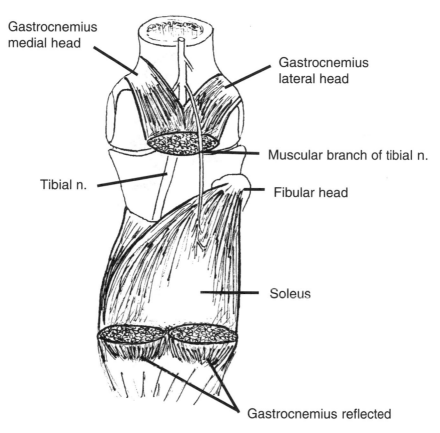

Gastrocnemius
medial head

Gastrocnemius
lateral head

Muscular branch of tibial n.

Tibial n.

Fibular head

Soleus

Gastrocnemius reflected

Figure 1A-31 The course of the tibial nerve in the posterior leg, between the two heads of the gastrocnemius and soleus, en route to the deep posterior leg.

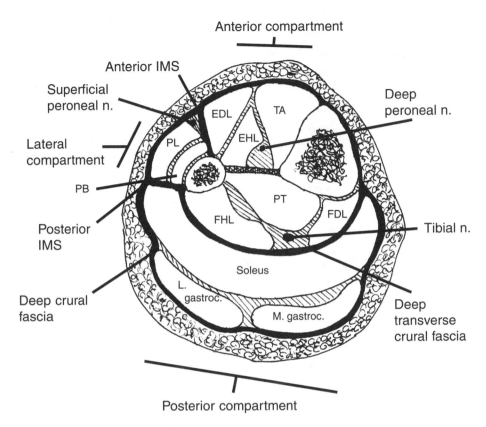

Figure 1A-32 Transverse section through the upper portion of the leg. The anterior compartment includes the tibialis anterior (TA), the extensor digitorum longus (EDL), and the extensor hallucis longus (EHL). The lateral compartment includes the peroneus longus (PL) and the peroneus brevis (PB). The posterior compartment contains the lateral gastrocnemius (L. gastroc.), the medial gastrocnemius (M. gastroc.), and the soleus superficially and the posterior tibialis (PT), the flexor digitorum longus (FDL), and the flexor hallucis longus (FHL) in the deep posterior compartment. (IMS = intermuscular septum.)

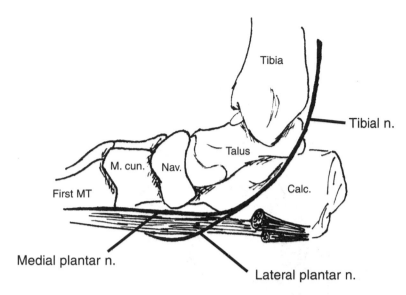

Figure 1A-33 The course of the tibial nerve posterior to the medial malleolus and subsequently into the foot, where it becomes the medial and lateral plantar nerves. (Calc. = calcaneus; Nav. = navicular; M. cun. = medial cuneiform; MT = metatarsal.)

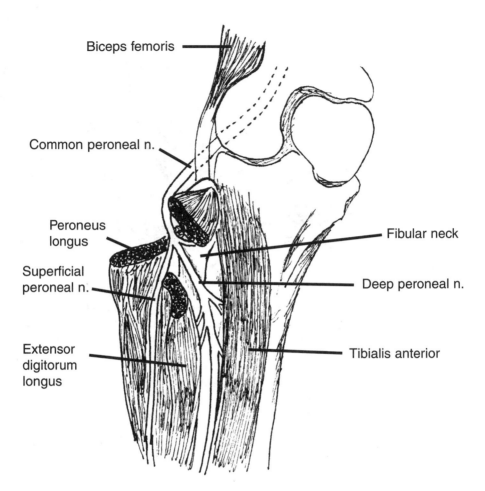

Figure 1A-34 Anterolateral view of the knee and proximal leg. Note the course of the common peroneal nerve around the fibular neck and its division into the superficial and deep peroneal nerves.

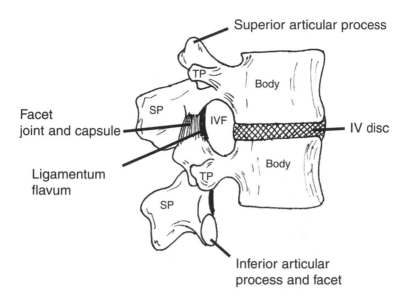

Figure 1A-35 Lateral view of a lumbar motion segment. Note the joints formed between the vertebrae, anteriorly between the bodies and posteriorly between the superior and inferior articular processes. Bordering the intervertebral foramen anteriorly are the bodies and disc; the pedicles are superior and inferior; and the facet joint, its capsule, and the ligamentum flavum are posterior. (SP = spinous process; TP = transverse process, IVF = intervertebral foramen; IV disc = intervertebral disc.)

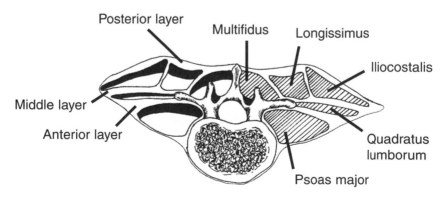

Figure 1A-36 Transverse section through the lumbar region. Note the trilaminar layer of the deep thoracolumbar fascia and the subsequent interconnections among the muscles of the low back.

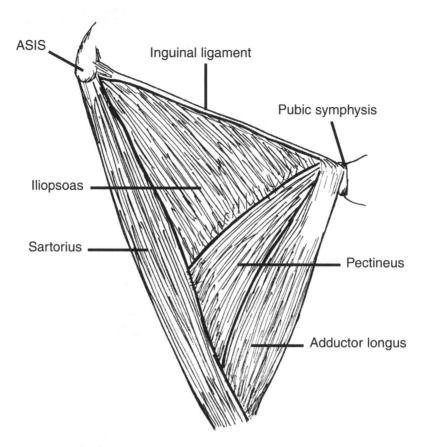

ASIS

Inguinal ligament

Pubic symphysis

Iliopsoas

Sartorius

Pectineus

Adductor longus

Figure 1A-37 The femoral triangle. The borders of the triangle are the sartorius laterally, the adductor longus medially, and the inguinal ligament superiorly. The floor of the femoral triangle is formed by the iliopsoas and pectineus. The contents of the femoral triangle (not shown) from lateral to medial are the femoral nerve, artery, vein, and lymph nodes. (ASIS = anterior superior iliac spine.)

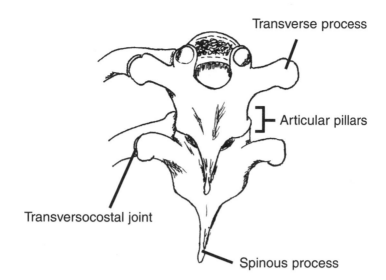

Figure 1A-38 Posterior view of a typical thoracic motion segment.

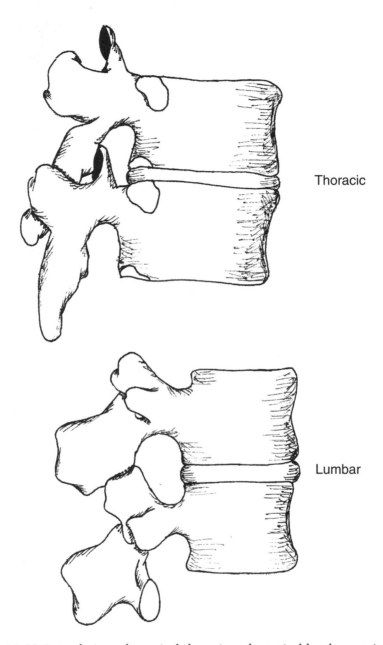

Thoracic

Lumbar

Figure 1A-39 Lateral view of a typical thoracic and a typical lumbar motion segment. Note the differences in the size, shape, and direction of the spinous processes.

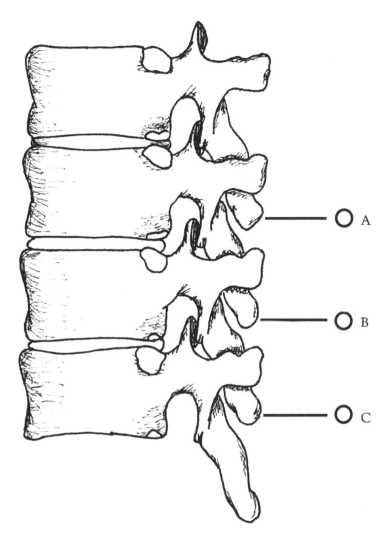

Figure 1A-40 Lateral view of the thoracic spine in normal sagittal plane alignment. Note the equivalent distances between points A, B, and C, representing the tips of adjacent spinous processes.

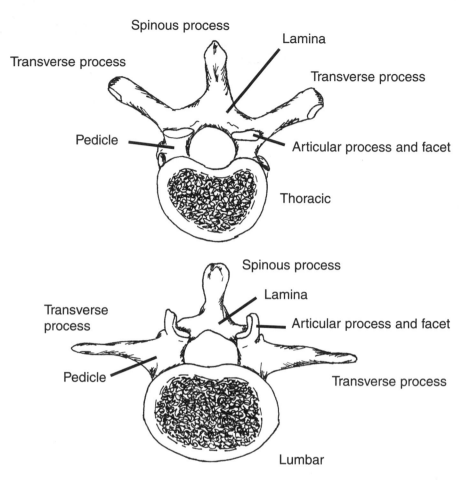

Figure 1A-41 Superior view of typical thoracic and lumbar vertebrae. Note the differences in the size, shape, and direction of the transverse processes.

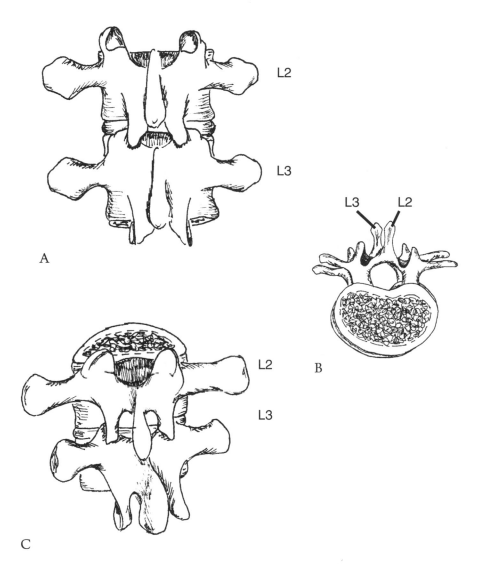

Figure 1A-42 (A) Posterior view of normally aligned lumbar vertebrae. Note the spinous processes are in line with one another. (B) Superior view of the L2–L3 motion segment in right rotation. Note the anterior position of the left transverse process and the posterior position of the right transverse process of the L2 vertebra. (C) Posterior view of the L2–L3 motion segment in right rotation. Note that the L2 spinous process is positioned to the left of the L3 spinous process (relatively). Positional faults are named according to the superior vertebra of the effected motion segment.

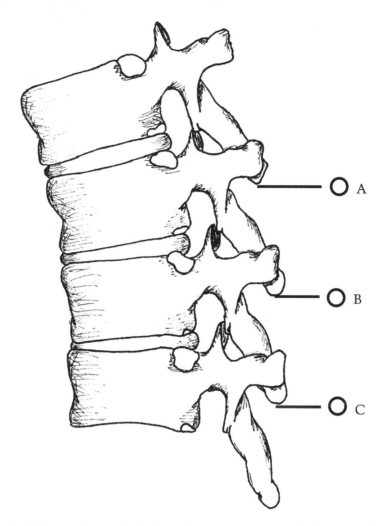

Figure 1A-43 Lateral view of the thoracic spine in a normally flexed position. Note the equivalent distances between points A, B, and C, representing the tips of adjacent spinous processes.

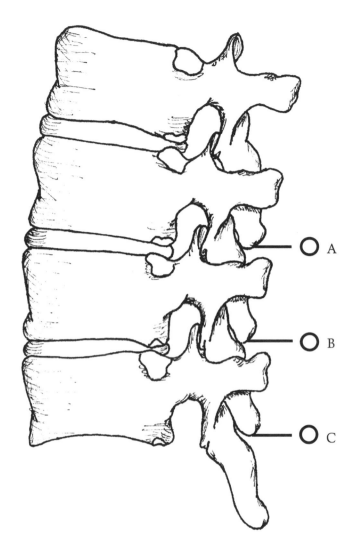

Figure 1A-44 Lateral view of the thoracic spine in a normally extended position. Note the equivalent distances between points A, B, and C, representing the tips of adjacent spinous processes.

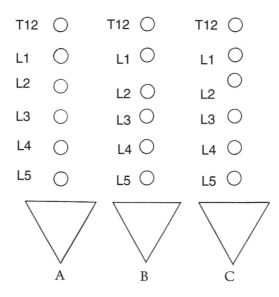

Figure 1A-45 Schematic of sagittal plane positional faults. The circles represent the tips of the spinous processes. The triangle represents the sacrum. (A) Normal sagittal plane position. (B) Extension of L2–3 segment. (C) Flexion of L2–L3 segment. The L2 vertebra was determined to be out of normal position because the distances between L1 and T12 and between L3 and L4 are symmetrical.

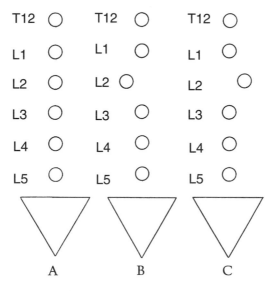

Figure 1A-46 Schematic of transverse plane positional faults. The circles represent the tips of the spinous processes. The triangle represents the sacrum. (A) Normal transverse plane position. (B) Right rotation of the L2–L3 segment. (C) Left rotation of the L2–L3 segment.

Superior articular process

Facet joint space

Inferior articular process

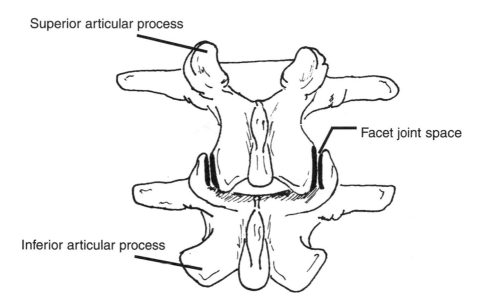

Figure 1A-47 Posterior view of the lumbar vertebrae. The facet joints are formed as adjacent inferior and superior articular processes articulate.

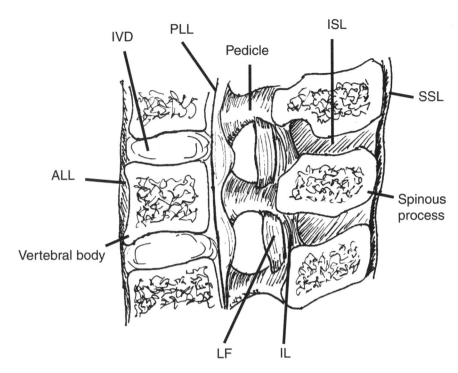

Figure 1A-48 Midsagittal section through the lumbar spine. (ALL = anterior longitudinal ligament; IVD = intervertebral disc; PLL = posterior longitudinal ligament; ISL = interspinous ligament; SSL = supraspinous ligament; IL = intrinsic ligaments of facet capsule; LF = ligamentum flavum.)

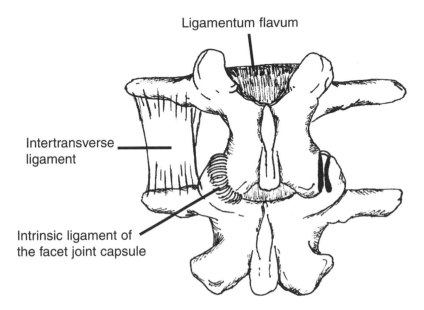

Ligamentum flavum

Intertransverse ligament

Intrinsic ligament of the facet joint capsule

Figure 1A-49 Posterior view of the lumbar vertebrae with some ligaments intact.

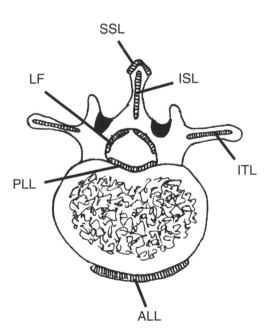

SSL

LF

ISL

ITL

PLL

ALL

Figure 1A-50 Superior view of the lumbar vertebrae with ligaments intact. (ALL = anterior longitudinal ligament; PLL = posterior longitudinal ligament; ISL = interspinous ligament; SSL = supraspinous ligament; LF = ligamentum flavum; ITL = intertransverse ligament.)

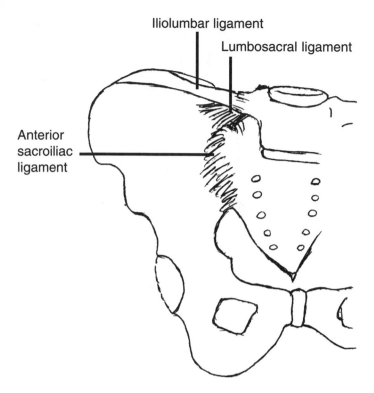

Figure 1A-51 Anterior view of the ligaments attaching the spine to the ilium and sacrum.

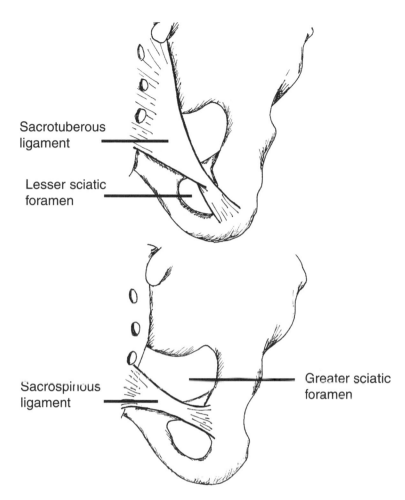

Figure 1A-52 Posterior view of the ligaments attaching the sacrum to the ischium.

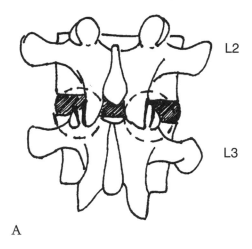

A

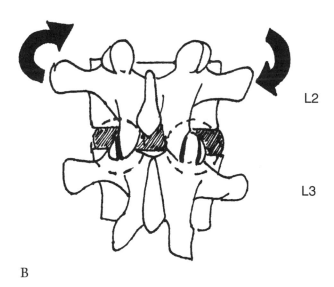

B

Figure 1A-53 Posterior view of lumbar facet joints. (A) Facet joint position with no rotation. (B) Facet joint position with right rotation of the L2–L3 motion segment. Note the "opening" of the right facet joint and the "closing" of the left facet joint.

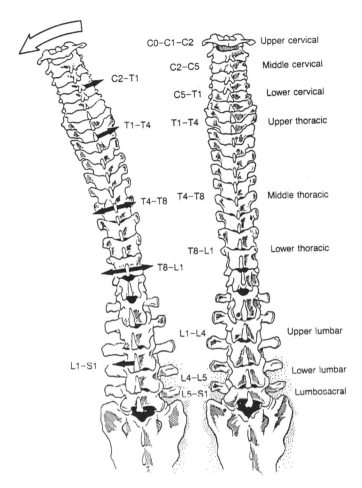

Figure 1A-54 Regional coupling patterns throughout the spine. This diagram summarizes the coupling of lateral bending and axial rotation and depicts the new biomechanical subdivisions of the spine. The actual coupling is between ± z-axis rotation and ± y-axis rotation. It can also be thought of in terms of the direction of movement of spinous processes with left lateral bending. Note that in the middle and lower cervical spine, as well as in the upper thoracic spine, the same coupling patterns are seen. In the middle and the lower thoracic spine, the axial rotation, which is coupled with lateral bending, can be in either direction, that is, it can be ± y-axis rotation. The direction of this axial rotation apparently varies between different specimens. In the lumbar spine there is –y-axis rotation associated with –z-axis rotation. That is, the spinous processes go to the left with left lateral bending. The same pattern is also present at the lumbosacral functional segmental unit. (Reprinted with permission from AA White, MM Panjabi. Clinical Biomechanics of the Spine [2nd ed]. Philadelphia: Lippincott, 1990;104.)

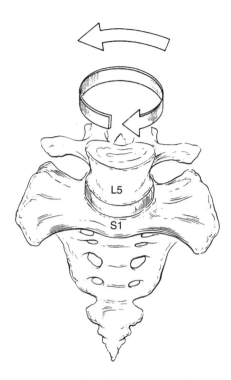

Figure 1A-55 L5–S1 rotation and sidebending coupling pattern. Rotation and ipsilateral sidebending are coupled at L5–S1. (Reprinted with permission from MM Panjabi, I Yamamoto, T Oxland, JJ Crisco. How does posture affect the coupling? Spine 1989;14:1002; and MJ Pearcy, SB Tibrewal. Axial rotation and lateral bending in the normal lumbar spine measured by three-dimensional radiography. Spine 1984;9:582.)

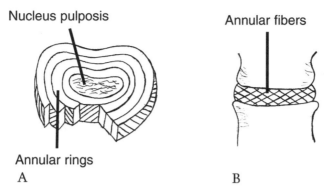

Nucleus pulposis

Annular fibers

Annular rings

A

B

Figure 1A-56 Intervertebral disc. (A) Superolateral view of a disc with part of the annular fibers cut away. The nucleus pulposus is surrounded by concentric rings (10–20 normally) of highly collagenous connective tissue. The fiber orientation of the concentric rings is alternating. (B) A lateral view of vertebral bodies joined by a vertebral disc. The schematic show fibers oriented in two directions, representing the consecutive layers of the annular fibers.

Appendix 1-2

Low Back Muscles*

Posterior Lumbar Spine Muscles

Erector Spinae Group (Sacrospinalis)

The proximal (inferior) attachment of this group of muscles is shared. The iliocostocervicalis, longissimus, and the spinalis muscles, which make up this group, inferiorly attach the median sacral crest, the spinous processes (SPs) of T11–L5 and their supraspinous ligaments, the medial aspect of the dorsal iliac crest, the lateral sacral crest, and the sacrotuberous and sacroiliac (SI) ligaments. Some fibers of this shared tendon blend with the gluteus maximus and multifidus.

Iliocostalis Lumborum

General attachments: common tendon to ribs
Proximal attachment (PA) (inferior): common tendon (see erector spinae group)
Distal attachment (DA) (superior): lower 6–7 ribs at the angles
Innervation: dorsal rami of corresponding levels
Actions: extends and ipsilaterally sidebends the spine

Iliocostalis Thoracis

General attachments: primarily ribs to ribs
PA (inferior): lower 6–7 ribs at the angles (medial to its lumborum DA)
DA (superior): upper 6 ribs at the angles, posterior portion of the C7 transverse process (TP)
Innervation: dorsal rami of corresponding levels
Actions: extends and ipsilaterally sidebends the spine

Longissimus Thoracis

General attachments: lumbar TPs to thoracic TPs
PA (inferior): common tendon (see erector spinae group), posterior aspects of the lumbar TPs and accessory processes, middle layer of the thoracolumbar fascia
DA (superior): tips of T1–12 TPs and lower 9–10 ribs between the tubercles and angles
Innervation: dorsal rami of corresponding levels
Actions: extends and ipsilaterally sidebends the spine

---

*Boldface with the innervation root levels indicates primary sources of innervation.

Transversospinalis Group

Generally this muscle group attaches TPs to the adjacent (sometimes more distal sites) vertebra's SPs. Generally, the more superficial a muscle in this group, the longer its fibers. This group consists of semispinalis, multifidus, and rotatores muscles. Only the multifidus is significantly developed in the lumbar spine.

Multifidus
General attachments: a more laterally located spinal landmark or soft tissue to a more superiorly located SP (midline)
PA (inferior): dorsal surface of the sacrum, aponeurosis of the erector spinae, posterior superior iliac spine, the dorsal SI ligaments, all lumbar mamillary processes, all thoracic TPs, and the articular processes of C4–C7
DA (superior): SP of a more superiorly located vertebrae
Innervation: dorsal rami of corresponding segments
Actions: extends and contralaterally rotates the spine

Segmental Lumbar Spine Muscles

Interspinalis
General attachments: adjacent SPs
PA (inferior): superior surface of SP
DA (superior): inferior surface of the SP immediately superior to it
Innervation: dorsal rami of corresponding levels
Actions: extends the spine

Intertransversarii
General attachments: adjacent TPs (specific attachments vary among spinal regions)
PA (inferior): superior surface of TP
DA (superior): inferior surface of the TP superior to it
Innervation: dorsal and ventral rami
Actions: ipsilaterally sidebends the spine

Muscles of the Posterior Abdominal Wall

Psoas Major

General attachments: lumbar spine to proximal femur
PA: L1–L5 TPs along their anterior and lower borders, bodies of T12–L5 and adjoining discs

DA: lesser trochanter of the femur
Innervation: branch from the L1–L3 ventral rami
Actions: open chain—flexes the hip, laterally rotates the hip; closed chain—flexes trunk

Psoas Minor

General attachments: vertebrae and discs to pubis
PA: sides of T12 and L1 vertebral bodies and adjoining disc
DA: pecten pubis, iliopectineal eminence and iliac fascia
Innervation: branch of L1 spinal nerve
Actions: weak trunk flexor

Iliacus

General attachments: ilium, ligaments, and sacrum to femur
PA: superior two-thirds of iliac fossa, inner lip of iliac crest, ventral SI and iliolumbar ligaments, and ala of sacrum
DA: lesser trochanter of femur and the area immediately anterior and inferior to it
Innervation: branch of femoral nerve (L2,3)
Actions: flexes the hip

Quadratus Lumborum

General attachments: ilium and ligament to rib
PA (inferior): iliolumbar ligament, posteromedial iliac crest (5 cm)
DA (superior): twelfth rib along the medial one-half of the lower border
Innervation: branch of T12–L3 (sometimes branches from L4) ventral rami
Actions: open chain—stabilizes the twelfth rib, laterally flexes trunk, bilaterally it may extend the trunk; closed chain—hikes the hip

Anterior Thigh Muscles Attaching to the Pelvis

Sartorius

General attachments: ilium to tibia
PA: Anterior superior iliac spine (ASIS), upper one-half of the notch inferior to ASIS
DA: proximal medial tibia at the pes anserine
Innervation: femoral nerve (L2,3)

Actions: flexes, externally rotates and abducts the hip, flexes and externally rotates the knee

Rectus Femoris

General attachments: ilium to quadriceps tendon
PA: straight head—anterior inferior iliac spine; reflected head—groove superior to acetabulum, fibrous capsule of hip joint
DA: patella by quadriceps tendon, tibial tuberosity by patellar tendon (ligament)
Innervation: femoral nerve (L2,**3**,**4**)
Actions: flexes the hip, extends the knee

Medial Thigh Muscles Attaching to the Pelvis

Gracilis

General attachments: pubis and ischium to tibia
PA: lower one-half of the pubic body, lower inferior pubic ramus and adjoining inferior ischial ramus
DA: proximal medial tibia at the pes anserine
Innervation: obturator nerve (**L2**,3)
Actions: flexes and medially rotates the knee and adducts the hip

Pectineus

General attachments: pubic bone to femur
PA: pecten pubis, pubic bone between the iliopectineal eminence and the pubic tubercle.
DA: a line on the posteromedial femur connecting the intertrochanteric line and the linea aspera
Innervation: femoral nerve (L2,**3**), accessory obturator nerve (L3)
Actions: adduction of the hip

Adductor Longus

General attachments: pubis to femur
PA: pubic body
DA: linea aspera within the middle one-third of the femur (between the attachments of vastus medialis and adductor magnus)
Innervation: obturator nerve (L2,**3**,**4**)
Actions: adducts the hip

Adductor Brevis

General attachments: pubis to femur
PA: lateral aspect of the pubic body, inferior pubic ramus between the PAs of gracilis and obturator externus
DA: posteromedial femur along a line connecting the lesser trochanter and the linea aspera
Innervation: femoral nerve (L2,**3**,**4**)
Actions: adducts the hip

Adductor Magnus

General attachments: pubis and ischium to femur
PA: small portion of pubic ramus (posterior portion), adjacent inferior ischial ramus, ischial tuberosity along its inferolateral aspect
DA: gluteal tuberosity medial to the gluteus maximus, linea aspera and proximal portion of the medial supracondylar line, adductor tubercle of the medial femoral condyle
Innervation: obturator nerve, tibial division of the sciatic nerve (L2,**3**,**4**)
Actions: adducts the hip, secondarily extends the hip

Posterior Thigh Muscles Attaching to the Pelvis

Biceps Femoris

General attachments: ischium and femur to fibula and ligament
PA: long head—upper ischial tuberosity along its inferomedial impression; short head—lateral lip of the linea aspera (lateral to adductor magnus and medial to vastus lateralis) inferior to the gluteus maximus attachment, connecting with the lateral supracondylar line 5 cm from the lateral femoral condyle
DA: fibular head, lateral collateral ligament of the knee, lateral tibial condyle
Innervation: long head—tibial division of the sciatic nerve (L5, **S1**,2)
Actions: extends the hip, flexes the knee, secondarily laterally rotates the hip and knee

Semitendinosus

General attachments: ischium to tibia
PA: upper ischial tuberosity along its inferomedial impression
DA: medial aspect of the proximal tibia

Innervation: tibial division of the sciatic nerve (**L5**, **S1**,2)
Actions: extends the hip, flexes the knee, secondarily medially rotates the hip and knee

Semimembranosus

General attachments: ischium to tibia
PA: upper ischial tuberosity along its superolateral impression
DA: posterior aspect of the medial tibial condyle
Innervation: tibial division of the sciatic nerve (**L5**, **S1**,2)
Actions: extends the hip, flexes the knee, secondarily medially rotates the hip and knee

Muscles of the Buttock

Gluteus Maximus

General attachments: ilium, sacrum, coccyx, and connective tissue to femur and iliotibial band (ITB)
PA: posterior gluteal line of the external surface of the ilium and the ilium posterosuperior to this including the crest, dorsal surface of lower sacrum, side of the coccyx, aponeurosis of erector spinae and the sacrotuberous ligament
DA: gluteal tuberosity of the femur and ITB
Innervation: inferior gluteal nerve (L5, **S1**,2)
Actions: extends, abducts, and laterally rotates the hip, stabilizes the knee through the action of the ITB

Gluteus Medius

General attachments: ilium to femur
PA (inferior): the external surface of the ilium in the area between the iliac crest, the posterior gluteal line and the anterior gluteal line and to the deep fascia covering its anterior aspect
DA (superior): lateral aspect of the greater trochanter of the femur
Innervation: superior gluteal nerve (**L5**, S1)
Actions: abduct and internally rotate the hip

Gluteus Minimus

General attachments: ilium to femur

PA: the external surface of the ilium in the area between the anterior gluteal line and to the inferior gluteal line, and from the margin of the greater sciatic notch
DA: anterolateral ridge on the greater trochanter of the femur
Innervation: superior gluteal nerve (**L5**, S1)
Actions: open chain—abducts and internally rotates the hip; closed chain—prevents Trendelenburg's sign

Deep Buttock Muscles
Piriformis

General attachments: sacrum and ilium to femur
PA (inferior): ventral surface of the sacrum between the foramina, the gluteal surface of the ilium near the posterior inferior iliac spine, and the capsule of the SI joint.
DA (superior): superior medial aspect of greater trochanter posterosuperior to the trochanteric fossa
Innervation: branch from L5, **S1**,2
Actions: externally rotate the extended hip, abduct the flexed hip

Obturator Internus

General attachments: internal pelvic surface to femur
PA (inferior): anterosuperior wall of lesser pelvic cavity (around most of the obturator foramen, the inferior rami of the pubis and ischium, the pelvic surface posteroinferior to the pelvic brim, the obturator membrane's internal surface)
DA (superior): medial surface of greater trochanter of femur anterosuperior to its fossa
Innervation: nerve to obturator internus L5, **S1**
Actions: externally rotates the extended hip, abducts the flexed hip

Gemellus Superior

General attachments: ischium to femur
PA (inferior): ischial spine along its dorsal aspect
DA (superior): medial aspect of the greater trochanter of the femur
Innervation: nerve to obturator internus L5, **S1**
Actions: externally rotates the extended hip, abducts the flexed hip

Obturator Externus

General attachments: external aspect of the anterior pelvic wall to femur
PA (inferior): external aspect of the anterior pelvic wall (external surface of the obturator membrane, adjacent bone of pubic and ischial rami and the lip of their pelvic aspects
DA (superior): medial aspect of the greater trochanter within the trochanteric fossa
Innervation: posterior branch of the obturator nerve (L3,4)
Actions: externally rotates the hips

Gemellus Inferior

General attachments: ischium to femur
PA (inferior): ischial tuberosity inferior to the groove for the obturator internus tendon
DA (superior): medial aspect of the greater trochanter of the femur
Innervation: nerve to quadratus femoris L5, S1
Actions: externally rotates the extended hip, abducts the flexed hip

Quadratus Femoris

General attachments: ischial tuberosity to femur
PA (inferior): ischial tuberosity along its upper external aspect
DA (superior): quadrate tubercle of the femur
Innervation: nerve to quadratus femoris L5, S1
Actions: externally rotates the femur

2

Diseases and Disorders Affecting the Low Back

Brian P. D'Orazio
and Paul L. Lysher

Low back pain (LBP) is the common denominator of many diseases and disorders. The genesis of LBP from multiple organ systems complicates its differential diagnosis. Although not intended to be an exhaustive text on pathology, this chapter explores diseases and disorders that may cause LBP. The chapter begins by examining the relationship between age-related spinal changes and degenerative changes induced by either disease or injury.

Aging and Degeneration of the Lumbar Spine

Intervertebral Disc: Properties of Normal Aging

At birth, the nucleus of the intervertebral disc is approximately 88% water, compared with 78% for the annulus. These values drop to 65% for the nucleus and 70% for the annulus in aged subjects.[1] The intervertebral disc is composed of type I and type II collagen. Type II collagen is present in the nucleus pulposus and in the inner laminar rings of the annulus fibrosus. Peripheral layers of the annulus contain type I collagen. Tensile strength is largely a product of the type I collagen with type II collagen being better suited for compression loading.[2] Proteoglycan aggregates are associated particularly with the nucleus pulposus. These molecules are negatively charged and possess strong hydrophilic properties. The loss of some glycosaminoglycans in the nucleus is likely responsible for the overall decrease in nuclear water content, as fewer molecules are available to bind water.[3,4]

After the third decade of life, Galante reported that tensile properties of the annulus fibrosus are unaltered in nondegenerative specimens.[4] Healthy intervertebral discs are unlikely to rupture as a result of compressive trauma; rather, injury occurs at the vertebral body end plate.[5] Disc injury can occur more easily in an already degenerative disc.[6]

Degenerative Intervertebral Disc

Degenerative changes occur most commonly at L4–L5 and L5–S1.[7] The mechanism for this change is unknown. Mechanical studies have demonstrated that torsional stresses on the disc can create tears in the annular rings; therefore, it has been postulated that torsional stresses are the primary traumatic mechanism.[6] Anatomically, it is known that the anterior annulus fibrosus is stiffer and possesses significantly better recovery properties than the posterior annulus.[4,6] Annular tensile strength is weakest centrally and laterally, which correlates well with the posterolateral area being a common site for lumbar disc failure.[8] The precise association between these intrinsic disc factors, changes in lumbar intervertebral pressures with movement, and disc degeneration remains unclear.

Degenerative discs are more compressible than normal discs. Hirsch and Nachemson reported that with a 40-kg axial load there was no difference in deformation between healthy and degenerative discs.[9] With a 400-kg load, however, there was a 2.0-mm deformation in the degenerative discs compared with a 1.5-mm change in a healthy disc.[9] Degenerative discs withstand less translation and movement because of the inability of the annulus to resist sheer stresses.[1,6] In later years, the process spontaneously restabilizes and the disc translates through a smaller range.[10] These translations are small and of doubtful clinical significance except in severely degenerated discs, although some clinicians ascribe great significance to the instability that arises as a result of degenerative disc changes.[11–14]

Degenerative changes primarily take place in the noninnervated layers of the disc; therefore, these changes have no direct potential to produce pain. If the degenerative changes create lesions in the outer annular rings, there is the possibility for pain. Studies to date generally show poor correlations between radiographic signs of disc degeneration and pain, except in the most severe cases.[15–17]

Intervertebral Disc Derangement

Derangement within the intervertebral disc resulting from either injury or degeneration is common. The nomenclature for these changes, however, is inconsistent. Brant-Zawadzki and Jensen point out that the general term "herniation" has created confusion because of its inconsistent use in the litera-

Table 2-1 Definition of Disc Derangements

Type of disc derangement	Definition
Bulging disc	Circumferential extension of disc material beyond the end plates, in a generalized and outwardly convex fashion
Protruded disc	A broad-based but asymmetric (noncircumferential) extension of disc material occurring from the interspace, the dimension of the broad base against the parent disc being the largest diameter of the extending component
Extruded disc	A focal, asymmetric extension of disc material from the interspace, occurring in a way that the largest diameter of the extending fragment is greater than the base of connection to the parent disc

Source: Quoted from M Brant-Zawadzki, M Jensen. Imaging corner spinal nomenclature. Spine 1995;20:388.

ture and its poor correlation between anatomic changes and symptoms.[18] They divide pathologic intervertebral disc changes into three categories: bulging disc, protruding disc, and extruded disc (Table 2-1). The authors note that few asymptomatic individuals are identified as having a disc extrusion, whereas the term *herniation* applies to a much larger population, probably owing to the frequently asymptomatic condition of a bulging or protruding disc.

Discitis

Discitis occurs as the result of an intervertebral disc infection. This is most commonly associated with an invasion of bacteria into the disc after intervertebral disc surgery, a disc space injection, or a discogram. Intervertebral discs can also become infected through other foci, such as a bacterial infection in the anterior vertebral body that secondarily invades the intervertebral disc. Urinary tract infections have been associated with infections of intervertebral discs.[19]

Posterior Elements

Age-related changes are considered a separate phenomenon from degeneration.[4] The ligamentum flavum, for example, retains its physical properties without morphologic changes during normal aging.[20,21] Changes in the posterior elements occur predominately as a result of changes in the intervertebral disc.[22]

Degenerative Changes in Zygapophyseal Joints

Degenerative changes in zygapophyseal joints generally do not appear until after age 30 years.[23] Lewin described three levels of degeneration in lumbar zygapophyseal joints (Table 2-2). In older adults, larger fat pads are associated with articular cartilage loss. These fat pads are innervated and therefore capable of nociception. Fibrocartilaginous inclusions, which may be the result of articular cartilage loose bodies attaching to the joint capsule, potentially impinge between the articular cartilage surfaces. These are thought to be painful as a result of pressure on the joint capsule.[24] Unfortunately, the role of these inclusions in producing LBP remains theoretical because there is no validated clinical test to evaluate their presence.

Lumbar motion segment mobility begins to diminish past age 12 years, but more dramatically beyond age 35 years.[24,25] The intervertebral disc is partially responsible; however, the relative contribution of the disc versus the posterior elements is not clearly delineated in the literature. Furthermore, the debate over zygapophyseal joint stability as associated with degenerative changes remains unresolved. Mobility diminishes dramatically through the zygapophyseal joints later in life, but during the middle years, when back pain is most common, mobility remains in question. Theories of zygapophyseal joint instability are largely attributable to osteophyte formation in the intervertebral joints. Some authors believe that these changes are the result of increased joint translation; however, most of these theories are anecdotal.[11,12,14,26]

Table 2-2 Lumbar Zygapophyseal Joint Degeneration

Classification	Description
Degree 1	The synovial membrane and articular capsule are not usually involved at this stage. There is peripheral loss of articular cartilage with occasional deep fissuring in the cartilage. Degree 1 changes typically appear after 20 years of age.
Degree 2	Small deposits of new bone are seen at the capsular attachments. The synovial and fibrous layers of the joint capsule are not clearly delineated and some thickening of the subchondral bone plate is evidenced. Necrotic areas are noted in the articular cartilage. This level is typically encountered at age 45.
Degree 3	Isolated osseous tissue is occasionally embedded in the connective tissue. There are large areas of articular cartilage destruction sometimes with evidence of fibrous tissue replacing the articular cartilage. These changes are usually not seen until age 60.

Source: Quoted from T Lewin. Osteoarthritis in lumbar synovial joints: a morphological study. Acta Orthop Scand 1994;73[Suppl].

Aging and Degeneration
of the Sacroiliac Joints

There do not appear to be any studies that separately view aging versus degeneration in the sacroiliac joints. Furthermore, there are no studies about this phenomenon at the pubic symphysis. Studies of mobility probably provide us with the best evidence of functional change in sacroiliac joints. In males older than age 30 years, 60% of sacroiliac joint specimens demonstrate osteophytes.[27] This percentage increases to 86% in the fourth decade of life and is 100% beyond age 50 years. Beyond age 50, 60% of male sacroiliac joints were considered to demonstrate ankylosis, with 50% demonstrating ankylosis from 40 to 49 years of age. These changes are slower to take place in most females; in women in their 40s, only 50% of sacroiliac joints demonstrate osteophytes and this rises to 86% for women in their 50s. For females, generally there were no specimens demonstrating ankylosis before age 50 years.

Many diseases have an expression in the sacroiliac joints. These include ankylosing spondylitis, pelvic tumors, rheumatoid arthritis, and others. The frequency of sacroiliac joint symptoms is uncertain. McKenzie stated, "disorders of the sacroiliac joint occur without doubt, but most are inflammatory in origin. It is also recognized that true mechanical lesions do occur. They are, however, uncommon and usually occur following pregnancy. Physical therapists, especially in the United States or wherever therapists are receiving instruction from osteopaths, are "discovering" sacroiliac joint pathology in many of their patients. It is likely that either their components are wrong or the literature is in error."[28] Schwarzer indicated that 30% of 43 subjects with complaints of LBP below the L5–S1 level experienced significant relief of symptoms when the sacroiliac joints were injected.[29] Reliability of sacroiliac joint testing, based on common tests, is poor, leaving unanswered the question of how to reliably examine and treat the sacroiliac joints.[30]

Structural Disorders

Schmorl's Nodes

First described by Schmorl in 1930, Schmorl's nodes are prolapses of disc material into the trabecular bone of the vertebral body. There are generally two types: peripheral and central. Central Schmorl's nodes are considered to be the most common and occur through the vertebral end plate as a result of a weakened area left by the embryonic notochord tract. Central nodes are usually considered to be asymptomatic. Peripheral nodes occur along vascular canals, again at weak points through the end plate.

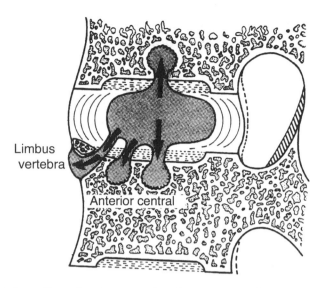

Figure 2-1 Schmorl's nodes. (Reprinted with permission from LT Twomey, JR Taylor [eds]. The Lumbar Spine from Infancy to Old Age. In Physical Therapy of the Low Back. New York: Churchill Livingstone, 1987;32.)

Anterior peripheral nodes are more common than posterior nodes and are often associated with trauma (Figure 2-1). Schmorl's nodes occur in 36% of adult spines in the lumbar and thoracic vertebra.[24.]

Spondylolysis and Spondylolisthesis

"Spondylolisthesis refers to the forward displacement of one vertebra on another. The condition is most commonly seen at the lumbosacral junction. Spondylolysis, a defect in the pars interarticularis is present in about 5–6% of the adult population."[31] Commonly, there are five broad etiologic classifications for spondylolisthesis and spondylolysis (Table 2-3). The most common classification in both children and adults younger than age 50 years is a type II lesion, termed "isthmic."[32] A spondylolysis may exist that is unilateral or bilateral but is defined by the lack of displacement of the vertebra. Its presence in the asymptomatic population is approximately equal to its prevalence in the patient population.[33] For many years, spondylolysis was assumed to be caused by an incomplete fusion of the neural arch at the pars interarticularis. Studies have demonstrated, however, that this defect does not exist in those individuals who have never been ambulatory, and furthermore, stress fractures have been demonstrated at the pars interarticularis in adolescents. This condition has been shown to occur

Table 2-3 Classification of Spondylolisthesis/Spondylolysis

Type	Description
I. Dysplastic	Congenital malformations of primarily the superior sacral facets or the vertebral arch of L5 allow the occurrence of olisthesis.
II. Isthmic	Common in both children and adults, this lesion or defect in the pars interarticularis allows anterior vertebral migration, typically of L5. Three types are commonly described: a. Lytic: resulting from a fatigue fracture of the pars interarticularis b. Elongated pars interarticularis: the pars interarticularis is intact c. Fracture
III. Degenerative	Secondary to long-standing segmental instability with joint degeneration. Occurs most frequently at L4–L5.
IV. Traumatic	Secondary to fractures not involving the pars interarticularis.
V. Pathologic	Local or generalized structural weakness secondary to bone disease.

Source: Adapted from LL Wiltse, PH Newman, I MacNab. Classification of spondylolysis and spondylolisthesis. Clin Orthop Rel Res 1976;117:23.

frequently in adolescent males and results from contact sports such as football. There seems to be little continuing support for the concept that this condition commonly is the result of a congenital defect.[33,34]

Spondylolisthesis exists more commonly in males than females and reportedly occurs 85–90% of the time at the L5–S1 level.[34–37] The contribution of spondylolisthesis to LBP remains controversial. Virta and Rönnemaa found no evidence of an increased association between mild to moderate spondylolisthesis—less than 50% vertebral displacement—and LBP (see Table 2-4 for grades of spondylolisthesis). Furthermore, they found no association between the vertebral level of spondylolisthesis and symptom severity.[37] Magora and Schwartz concluded that among occupational subjects, spondylolisthesis may predispose the subject to a greater risk of LBP both in frequency and severity.[33] Their conclusions, however, were not statistically supported because of low patient numbers in the spondylolisthesis group. Sato and Kikuchi concluded that a "functional prognosis" in patients with radiographic lumbar instability does not depend on the existence or type of radiographic instability. Rather, it depends primarily on the anatomic profile of the lateral recesses of the spinal canal.[38] Nonsurgical treatment is the accepted standard of care for adult isthmic spondylolisthesis with surgery being reserved for those with intractable low back pain or leg pain. Unfortunately, there seems to be no standard of care that is widely accepted for conservative treatment of patients with spondylolisthesis.[32]

Table 2-4 Grading of Spondylolisthesis

Grade	Description
I	Less than 25% of the vertebral body is displaced in relationship to the adjacent vertebra.
II	25–50% of the vertebra is displaced in relationship to the adjacent anterior vertebral body.
III	50–75% of the vertebra is displaced in relationship to the adjacent anterior vertebral body.
IV	More than 75% of the vertebra is displaced.

Source: Adapted from HW Meyerding. Spondylolisthesis. Surg Gynecol Obstet 1932;54:371–377.

Clinical examination sometimes reveals spondylolisthesis through the relative absence of a palpable spinous process or, in the case of a retrolisthesis, a relative prominence of a spinous process. The presence of a "lumbosacral dimple"[37] will sometimes provide visual evidence of a spondylolisthesis. If changes in posture create large variations in the clinician's ability to palpate the spinous process, the defect requires further radiographic study to quantify the instability. Recommended radiographic procedures include static films, dynamic sagittal plane films, or, as suggested by Friberg, traction-compression radiography.[36]

Spina Bifida Occulta

Spina bifida occulta is a congenital anomaly in which the neural arch is incompletely formed and there is either a partial or complete absence of the spinous process. Among 1,244 subjects with spina bifida occulta, Magora and Schwartz reported that 83% had involvement at S1, while in the remaining 17% it was at L5.[39] No subjects had involvement above L5. Furthermore, spinal bifida occulta was not found to be associated with LBP in this study.

Idiopathic Scoliosis

Scoliosis can be divided into the categories of functional and structural. Functional scoliosis is usually the result of a leg length inequality (see Chapter 4). The second type of scoliosis is termed *idiopathic structural scoliosis*. Twomey and Taylor reported that asymmetric growth, especially of the vertebral arch, is responsible for the development of scoliosis in an unspecified number of cases.[24] They also acknowledge, however, that other causes may operate in the etiology of structural scoliosis. A long-term follow-up of 219 patients with untreated adolescent idiopathic scoliosis was undertaken by Weinstein et al.[40] "Backache" was found to be more common in the scoliotic patients than in the general population, although it was never "disabling." LBP was "unrelated to the presence of osteoarthritic changes on roentgenogram." There was no correlation between the type and severity of curve and back symptoms. Thoracic curves measuring between 50 and 80 degrees and lumbar components of combined curves between 50 and 74 degrees tended to progress slightly in adult life. Pulmonary function was affected in patients with thoracic curves.[40]

Connolly et al.[41] evaluated 83 patients in whom adolescent idiopathic scoliosis had been treated with a posterior spinal arthrodesis and Harrington instrumentation extending to the second, third, fourth, or fifth lumbar vertebra. Sixty-three (76%) of these patients had a significant increase in LBP compared with 30 (50%) of 60 control individuals. The preoperative Cobb angle of the primary curve averaged 60 degrees and was an average of 35 degrees at the time of follow-up evaluation. Patients in whom the arthrodesis had extended to the lumbar segments had a significantly increased prevalence of degenerative changes.[41]

Asymmetries of the Vertebral Column

Vertebral column symmetry is considered the exception rather than the rule.[42] Most asymmetries are of no consequence except when misinterpreted as indicating underlying mechanical dysfunction. A common congenital anomaly is the midline deviation of thoracic spinous processes. These deviations can be interpreted as rotational dysfunctions, leading the clinician to manipulate a normal motion segment.[42]

The functional beginning of the lumbar spine varies considerably. In some individuals this occurs at the T10–T11 segment, although in many the transition is at T11–T12 or T12–L1. The transitional level is noted by the sagittal orientation of the articular facets. At the thoracolumbar junction, an extra rib attaching to the first lumbar vertebra is reported to have an incidence of 7.75%.[42]

Another common variation is asymmetry of the facet plane. Farfan and Sullivan reported that facet asymmetries predicted the level of disc herniation in a significant number of cases.[43] By contrast, Vanharanta and colleagues studied 106 patients using computed tomographic discography at

324 levels and reported, "There was no difference in degree of disc degeneration or pain response with respect to the facet tropism."[44]

At the lumbosacral junction many variations are reported. Sacralization or lumbarization of the last vertebra is common, causing lumbar vertebra to be numbered at between four and six. At L5, transverse processes are typically large and in some cases articulate either bilaterally or unilaterally with the sacrum, forming an adventitious joint. The transverse processes can also partially or completely fuse to the sacrum.[45]

Numerous anomalies exist in spinal neuroanatomy. A complete discussion is beyond the scope of this text; however, for surgeons the most significant anomaly may be intersegmental anastomosis. Because of this anomaly, localization of involvement is more complicated.[42]

A wide range of pelvic asymmetries exists, with Grieve reporting that "sacroiliac joint asymmetry is so common as to be the normal state."[42] Some of these asymmetries include accessory sacroiliac joints; asymmetrical formations of the sacrum; varying degrees of sacral agenesis; congenital widening of the symphysis pubis; extra bony prominences on the posterior surface of the iliac bones (Fong's disease, or iliac horn syndrome); variations in coccygeal angle, length, and formation; and leg length inequalities from a variety of sources along with many soft-tissue anomalies. These further complicate examination in this region.[42]

Spinal Stenosis

Spinal stenosis can be either developmental (congenital) or acquired. In developmental spinal stenosis, the vertebral canal is abnormally small, creating an environment that allows little room for the cauda equina. Amundsen and colleagues reported, "Much used normal values for the sagittal diameter (measured on the contrast column) is 13–20 mm (increasing caudally, though with a slight decrease at the fourth L4–5 level), the interpedicular distance 23–30 mm (also increasing caudally) and the pedicle length 3–10 mm (decreasing caudally)."[46] Congenital spinal stenosis is significant because relatively small changes in the central or lateral canal can be enough to compress the cauda equina. Acquired spinal stenosis is the result of hypertrophic changes in the spinal canal usually caused by combinations of degenerative disc disease and zygapophyseal osteoarthritis. In most cases of spinal stenosis, the clinical presentation includes lumbar pain in addition to sciatica, claudication symptoms related to walking, and pain that is usually reduced with slight forward bending. Amundsen et al., however, reported that some subjects in their study felt relief with extension that corresponded with an increase in vertebral canal sagittal plane diameter when those subjects extended.[46]

Connective Tissue Disease of the Spine

Ankylosing Spondylitis

Ankylosing spondylitis, which is more common in males, is characterized by widespread inflammatory disease of the vertebral column and sacroiliac joints with development of bony bridges between vertebrae. The initial presentation is a widening of the sacroiliac joints with subsequent fibrosis and sclerosis of subchondral bone. Hypomobility and eventual ankylosis then progress to include the vertebral motion segments.[47] Extremity joint involvement typically includes the hips, knees, and shoulders. These joints may become fibrotic or fuse, often with deformities. Chest expansion is reduced secondary to costovertebral joint involvement.[48]

Scheuermann's Disease

Scheuermann's disease, sometimes called osteochondrosis of the spine, is characterized by the presence of multiple Schmorl's nodes, anterior "wedging" of the vertebral bodies with a resultant thoracic kyphosis, irregular vertebral end plates, and narrowing of the intervertebral disc. Usually occurring during adolescence, the disease may exist asymptomatically in less severe cases.[24]

Reiter's Syndrome

Usually associated with urethritis and conjunctivitis, Reiter's syndrome is most commonly an adult male arthritic condition.[49] This triad of symptoms is a reactive process to an infectious agent.[50] The onset of arthritis may be acute or subacute.[49] Involvement is usually asymmetric and polyarticular, with a predilection for the feet, ankles, knees, and sacroiliac joints.[49,50] The arthritis tends to persist after the urethritis and conjunctivitis subside, affecting the spine and sacroiliac joints.[49]

Rheumatoid Arthritis

Rheumatoid arthritis is characterized by systemic disease, including synovitis and connective tissue inflammation, especially of the wrists, and proximal interphalangeal and metacarpal phalangeal joints of the hands. The physical therapist should be aware of axial instability when treating the cervical spine of patients with rheumatoid arthritis. Involvement of the lumbar spine and sacroiliac joints is not common, and LBP cannot usually be ascribed to rheumatoid inflammation.[51]

Fibromyalgia

Although not identifiable through any form of serologic testing, this syndrome is often considered to be a form of connective tissue disease characterized by the presence of trigger points in all quadrants, disturbed sleep patterns, and varying degrees of disability. Borenstein classified this syndrome into primary and secondary fibromyalgia.[52] Primary fibromyalgia is defined by the absence of other identifiable illnesses while still meeting the general definition for the syndrome. Secondary fibromyalgia is diagnosed when other disorders are present such as "postoperative states," lumbosacral arthritis, intervertebral disc herniation, or spinal trauma.[52] Treatment usually includes antidepressants to help the patient sleep and to reduce pain. Other treatments include muscle relaxants and cryotherapy, although heat is sometimes beneficial. Trigger point injections, various forms of soft-tissue treatment, and the short-term use of modalities to relieve pain also assist in achieving specific exercise goals. Patient education, psychological support if required, and involvement in support groups are important for a patient with this frustrating syndrome.

Polymyositis

The diagnosis of polymyositis is applied to any idiopathic condition in which there is inflammatory cell infiltration of muscle tissue. This may result in interstitial edema with muscle fiber necrosis and regeneration. When accompanied by skin manifestations, it is termed *dermatomyositis*.[53] Polymyositis may occur as a component of rheumatoid arthritis, scleroderma, or systemic lupus erythematosus and symmetrically affects the pelvic and shoulder girdle musculature.[48]

Psoriatic Arthritis

Psoriasis may develop into arthritis that is similar but clinically distinct from rheumatoid arthritis. Skin changes usually precede joint symptoms. These symptoms may simulate the appearance of gout, commonly affecting the distal interphalangeal joint of a finger or toe. Characterized by periods of exacerbation and remission, severe transient migratory "aches and pains" may develop in the spine.[48]

Paget's Disease

Paget's disease (osteitis deformans) is a common skeletal affliction with an unknown etiology that usually occurs in men older than age 50 years. There are several phases of osteoblastic destruction and repair, frequently involving the pelvis, femur, skull, tibia, and spine. The initial complaint is usually intermittent or constant pain (dull ache) in the area of bony involvement. The most common complication is fracture of a weight-bearing bone. LBP is commonly experienced with the eventual development of both a lumbar and thoracic kyphosis. Vertebral involvement can lead to compression of intraspinal structures and subsequent neurologic deficits.[48] In a retrospective study of 84 patients by Lander and Hadjipavlou,[54] nine developed pagetic intradiscal invasion from the adjacent vertebral bodies. This process may eventually produce ankylosis across a disc space.[54]

Polymyalgia Rheumatica

Characterized by complaints of bilateral pain and stiffness in the shoulder and pelvic girdle regions, the etiology of polymyalgia rheumatica is unknown.[53] Usually affecting those older than age 50 years, symptoms include muscular pain without joint swelling, an accompanying low-grade fever, and "malaise." Pain is usually worse in the morning or after extended sitting. Prolonged symptoms lead to disuse atrophy and weakness.[51,53]

Urogenital System

Female Conditions

Diseases or pathologic processes of the female urogenital organs can result in low back, pelvic, abdominal, or sacral referred pain (Table 2-5).[55]

It is important for clinicians to recognize pathologic signs and symptoms of common gynecologic and pregnancy conditions. Table 2-6 should assist in developing appropriate questions to be asked during history taking of female patients with urogenital signs and symptoms.[55]

Pelvic Inflammatory Disease

Pelvic inflammatory disease is typically an infection of the uterus, fallopian tubes, and broad ligaments caused by sexually transmitted disease.[55] Common symptoms include vaginal discharge, dysuria, low-grade fever, bilateral lower pelvic pain, LBP, and referred shoulder pain.[51] Rebound tenderness can be elicited with a sudden release of manual pressure to the abdomen.

Adhesions may develop after acute infection causing chronic pelvic pain.[55] Prolonged psoas irritation may lead to a hip flexor contraction and pain.[56] Pelvic inflammatory disease should be suspected in a young woman

Table 2-5 Referred Pain: Female Urogenital System

Structure	Segmental innervation	Potential site of referred pain
Ovaries	T10–T11	Lower abdomen, low back
Uterus	T10–L1	Lower abdomen, low back
Fallopian tubes	T10–L1	Lower abdomen, low back
Perineum	S2–S4	Sacral apex, suprapubic, rectum
External genitalia	L1–L2, S3–S4	Lower abdomen, medial anterior thigh, sacrum
Kidney	T10–L1	Ipsilateral low back and upper abdomin
Urinary bladder	T11–L2, S2–S4	Thoracolumbar, sacrococcygeal, suprapubic
Ureters	T11–L2, S2–S4	Groin, upper and lower abdomen, suprapubic, anterior-medial thigh, thoracolumbar

Source: Reprinted with permission from WG Boissonnault. Examination in Physical Therapy: Screening for Medical Diseases. New York: Churchill Livingstone, 1991;149.

(ages 15–25 years) whose pelvic or low back symptoms are unchanged by either position or activity.[51] There should be careful questioning about any changes in menstrual cycle symptoms.

Endometriosis

In the United States, endometriosis most commonly occurs in white women between the ages of 25 and 45 years.[51] Tissue from the endometrium is typically found in the pelvic cavity, peritoneum, ovaries, rectum, and around the fallopian tubes.[55] The classic triad of symptoms is dysmenorrhea (painful menstruation), dyspareunia (painful intercourse), and infertility. Pain may be localized centrally in the sacrum, bilateral lower abdominal, or thigh regions. It may also be present in the lower thoracic or shoulder girdle area.[51] Pain begins in the premenstrual phase and continues during menstruation. Endometriosis may also involve the uterosacral ligaments or sacral plexus and may become a source of chronic LBP.[56,57]

Infections of the Bladder

Acute bacterial cystitis is an infection of the urinary bladder characterized by irritative voiding symptoms, including frequency, urgency, nocturia, burning on urination, and dysuria. Low back and suprapubic pain are also common complaints. The use of short-term antimicrobial therapy is usually effective in treating uncomplicated cystitis in women.[58]

Table 2-6 Female Urogenital System Checklist

Sign/symptom	Yes	No	Comments
1. Dyspareunia			
2. Dysmenorrhea			
3. Amenorrhea			
4. Abnormally heavy menstrual bleeding			
5. Abnormal bleeding pattern			
6. Vaginal discharge			
7. Vaginal burning/itching			
8. Dysuria			
9. Urinary frequency			
10. Urinary urgency			
11. Urinary incontinence			
12. Abdominal pain not associated with menstruation			
13. Abdominal bloating			
14. Postural hypotension			
15. History of infertility			
16. History of infection			

Source: Reprinted with permission from WG Boissonnault. Examination in Physical Therapy: Screening for Medical Disease. New York: Churchill Livingstone, 1991;149.

Ectopic Pregnancy

Ectopic pregnancy occurs when the fertilized ovum becomes implanted outside the uterus, usually in a fallopian tube.[56] There may be a history of previous pelvic infection or menstrual irregularity. The onset of pain is sudden, located either unilaterally or bilaterally in the lower abdomen with referral to the low back or shoulders.[51,55] Prompt medical attention is mandated.

Normal Pregnancy

Clinicians should be aware of the signs and symptoms of normal pregnancy listed in Table 2-7.

The release of the hormones relaxin and progesterone during pregnancy increases the laxity of the sacroiliac and other pelvic girdle ligaments to facilitate childbirth. This process leads to hypermobility of the pubic, sacroiliac, and sacrococcygeal joints, contributing to the development of an

Table 2-7 Signs and Symptoms of Normal Pregnancy

1. Nausea and vomiting

2. Frequent urination

3. Supine hypotension

4. Posture and mobility changes

5. Low back and hip pain (increases with size of fetus)

6. Thoracic outlet syndrome

7. Carpal tunnel syndrome

8. Edema in hands/feet

9. Breast tenderness

10. Fatigue

11. Dyspnea

Source: Reprinted with permission from FW Ling, PM King, CA Myers. Screening for Female Urogenital System Disease. In WG Boissonnault (ed), Examination in Physical Therapy Practice: Screening for Medical Disease. New York: Churchill Livingstone, 1991;135.

anterior pelvic tilt and increased lumbar lordosis.[55,59] There has been considerable debate in the literature over the causative relationship between lumbar lordosis and LBP. In a study by Fast and colleagues in 1986,[60] more than 50% of 200 women interviewed reported LBP during the fifth and seventh months of pregnancy. One theory is that the rapidly developed lordotic posture may alter the load distribution in the motion segment and place an excessive demand on the trunk musculature. "The overstretched abdominal muscles and the shortened back muscles are at a mechanical disadvantage and may not be able to withstand the demands imposed by the postural changes and excessive loads."[60] Excessive stress may be placed on the zygapophyseal joints as a result of the anterior shift in the center of gravity.[59] These postural changes may also cause sacroiliac or hip pain.[55] A lumbar support, gentle stretching exercises, cryotherapy, and education in postural adjustments can be helpful in alleviating symptoms.[59]

Hormonal Dysfunction

Stress or a failure of complex neuroendocrine feedback loops can cause irregular and unpredictable menstrual cycles. Endocrine abnormalities caused by thyroid, adrenal, or pituitary dysfunction can also affect ovulation and potentially lead to premature menopause. Menopause occurs when the ovaries cease to produce estrogen, which can result in osteoporosis and thereby increase the risk of pathologic fractures to either the thoracic or lumbar vertebrae.[55]

Fibroids

Fibroids are benign muscle tumors usually found in the uterus. They are most prevalent in black women of reproductive age. Symptoms include menorrhagia (heavy menstrual bleeding), metrorrhagia (irregular bleeding), and intermenstrual bleeding. Large fibroid tumors can cause chronic pelvic pain and pressure symptoms to the bladder or rectum with occasional referral to the low back or sacral region.[55]

Cancer

Carcinoma of the uterine cervix ranks third in frequency after breast and skin cancers. Late symptoms may include LBP as a result of compression of lumbosacral nerves, direct involvement of lumbosacral nerve roots, pressure from a large tumor, or, occasionally, urethral obstruction.[61] Uterine carcinoma (body or cervix) may invade the uterosacral ligaments, causing localized sacral pain below the lumbosacral junction.[57] The peak incidence of ovarian carcinomas is in women in their late 50s. Detection is difficult until the neoplasm enlarges or extends enough to produce symptoms. Early symptoms may include vague lower abdominal discomfort and mild digestive complaints. Advanced malignancies may present with swelling of the abdomen.[49] Ovarian tumors may also become symptomatic if they rupture, twist, or bleed.[55] A postmenopausal patient with bleeding should be referred for evaluation of the reproductive system for malignancy.

Male Conditions

Diseases of the male urogenital organs can result in low back, pelvic, or hip symptoms ranging from a dull ache to a burning sensation or "wave-like" pain depending on the involved structure.[62] Questions pertaining to bladder or sexual function (Table 2-8) can provide valuable information regarding the health of the urogenital system.[62]

"Right and left upper quadrant abdominal pain can reflect ipsilateral renal and proximal ureter abnormalities."[62] Likewise, lower quadrant abdominal pain can be caused by ipsilateral distal ureteral, testicular, and epididymis disease.[62] Bladder disease pain may be referred to any area of the lower abdomen.

Bladder Cancer

The highest incidence of bladder cancer occurs in white males older than age 30 years who smoke. It is the fifth most common

Table 2-8 Review of Systems Checklist: Male Urogenital System

Sign/symptom	Yes	No	Comments
1. Dysuria			
2. Hematuria			
3. Incontinence			
4. Frequency of urination			
5. Urinary urgency			
6. Decreased force of urinary flow			
7. Impotence			
8. Pain with ejaculation			
9. Difficulties with maintaining an erection			
10. Urethral discharge			
11. History of urinary infection			
12. History of venereal disease			

Source: Reprinted with permission from WG Boissonnault. Examination in Physical Therapy: Screening for Medical Disease. New York: Churchill Livingstone, 1991;127.

cause of cancer death in men.[62] The most common symptoms include hematuria, dysuria, nocturia, and urinary urgency. Most bladder tumors are malignant, with metastases to the lungs, bones, and liver.[62] Patients with advanced bladder cancer may present with pelvic pain caused by an enlarging tumor mass or a nerve root irritation.[63]

Prostate Cancer

Prostate gland carcinoma is the third leading cause of cancer in men usually older than age 50 years. There are usually no overt signs or symptoms in the early stages of this disease. The first symptom may be a complaint of a "dull diffuse ache" localized to the central lower lumbar spine or upper sacral area. As the tumor grows, urinary dysfunction will be noted by the patient. Sites of metastasis include the lumbar and thoracic spine, the pelvis, the proximal femur, the ribs, and the sternum.[64]

Prostatitis and Prostatodynia

Prostate infections can typically cause low back, sacral, and perineal pain in younger (ages 20–30 years) or older (ages 50–60 years) men. Usually there are associated urinary symptoms. Patients with symptoms of prostatodynia may have pain in the perineum, pelvis, or low back, suggesting

Table 2-9 Structures of the Male Urogenital System

Structure	Segmental innervation	Possible areas of pain referral
Kidney	T10–L1	Lumbar spine (ipsilateral) flank; upper abdominal
Ureter	T11–L2, S2–S4	Groin; upper/lower abdominal; suprapubic, scrotum; medial, proximal thigh; thoracolumbar
Urinary bladder	T11–L2, S2–S4	Sacral apex; suprapubic; thoracolumbar
Prostate gland	T11–L1, S2–S4	Sacral, low lumbar; testes; thoracolumbar
Testes	T10–T11	Lower abdominal; sacral

Source: Reprinted with permission from WG Boissonnault. Examination in Physical Therapy: Screening for Medical Disease. New York: Churchill Livingstone, 1991;124.

prostatitis, but there are no objective findings of prostate inflammation or urinary tract infection.[64] Bladder disorders, stress, and emotional problems may be associated with this syndrome.[58] Table 2-9 shows the possible areas of pain referred from the various urogenital structures.[62]

Conditions Common to Both Male and Female Urogenital Systems

Pyelonephritis

Acute pyelonephritis, an inflammatory process of the renal parenchyma, is the most common renal disease encountered after an untreated bladder infection. This condition should be considered in diabetic patients, cancer patients undergoing chemotherapy, or in those patients who have had recent instrumented urinary diagnostic procedures.[62] Pain is described as a dull constant ache usually located in the ipsilateral lumbar spine with frequent radiation to the lower abdominal regions.[51,62] Examination of the musculoskeletal structures in this same region should help in making a differential diagnosis.[62]

Chronic Renal Failure

Chronic renal failure is characterized by progressive loss of nephrons resulting from a multitude of pathologic causes. Chronic renal failure may lead to increased bone resorption secondary to elevated levels of parathyroid hormone. Local pain complaints may result from microtrauma to bone resulting from decreased bone density. The vertebral column and femurs are most commonly involved.[62] Extreme caution must be taken during manual evaluation and treatment of these patients to reduce the risk of fracture.[51] Over time, there is irreversible loss of kidney function associated with the accumulation of nitrogenous wastes. Neurologic changes not associated with a specific dermatomal or myotomal pattern may develop. Common neurologic changes include increased deep tendon reflexes, intermittent paresthesias and hyperesthesias of the hands and feet, cramping of limb musculature, and absence of sweating.[62]

Urinary Stones

Calculi, or stones, may occur anywhere in the urinary tract, and symptoms depend on the location of the obstruction. LBP can be experienced when stones obstruct one or more calices, the renal pelvis, or the proximal ureter. Distal ureteral stones in males cause pain to radiate along the inguinal canal into the groin and testicle. In females, the pain may be referred to the labia.[58]

Gastrointestinal Disorders

Pathologic conditions of the gastrointestinal symptoms can lead to symptoms of low back, thoracic spine, or lower extremity pain. It is imperative that clinicians be able to identify signs and symptoms of visceral disease that may either coexist or be the primary cause of spinal complaints. It is interesting to note the relationship of the gastrointestinal organs to the musculoskeletal system. The duodenum is the first 25 cm of the small intestine, located in the right upper quadrant and almost entirely in the retroperitoneal area. It lies on top of the psoas major and courses across the vertebral column at the level of L4.[65] The ascending and descending colon are also retroperitoneal structures in the abdominal cavity that lie on top of the right iliacus and quadratus lumborum and in the angle between the left psoas major and quadratus lumborum, respectively.[66]

Acid Peptic Disorders

Acid peptic disorders are a common pathologic condition of the stomach and the first part of the duodenum and include reflux esophagitis, gastritis, gastric ulcer, duodenitis, and duodenal ulcer.[65] The classic pathologic feature is damage to the mucosa caused by an imbalance of acid, pepsin, bicarbonate, and mucus production of the intestinal tract.[51,65] Patients may complain of lower thoracic (i.e., thoracolumbar junction), upper abdominal, or anterior rib pain described as a "gnawing" sensation that is worse at night or when the stomach is empty. Heavy smoking or alcohol use and the intake of nonsteroidal anti-inflammatory drugs increase the incidence of acid peptic disorders.[65] As mentioned previously, it is important to obtain this information in the patient history.[67]

Hepatitis and Cholecystitis

Hepatitis (inflammation of the liver) and cholecystitis (inflammation of the gallbladder) can refer pain to the right upper abdominal quadrant, right posterior thoracic region, or shoulder region. Pain is usually abrupt in onset and is accompanied by nausea, vomiting, and fever. With patients who exhibit these symptoms, it is recommended that a baseline temperature be taken. Obese females older than age 40 years have the highest incidence of cholecystitis.[65]

Pancreatitis

Inflammation of the pancreas is caused by alcohol abuse (40%), gallstones (40%), or idiopathic causes (20%).[51] One-half of patients with pancreatitis will have pain radiating to the upper lumbar and lower thoracic area in addition to the mid-epigastric and left upper abdominal quadrant. The pain is constant in behavior and intensifies with eating, alcohol intake, and vomiting.[51,65]

Diverticulitis

Diverticulitis is a local inflammation in the wall of the apex of the "small intestinal pouch" caused by trapped fecal material.[49,51] Diverticulitis frequently presents in the descending or sigmoid colon, causing constant lower abdominal pain that may radiate to the low back, pelvis, or hip.[65] In patients older than age 40 years who present with hip or sacroiliac joint disease, it is important to determine whether presenting complaints are due to biomechanical dysfunction or to diverticulitis.[51] Again, changes in bowel function must be ascertained.[67]

Enlargement of the Spleen

Left upper abdominal pain, middle LBP, or left LBP can be caused by an enlarged spleen secondary to cancer, mononucleosis, or sickle cell disease. The most serious complication can be splenic rupture, which can lead to massive bleeding and death. Soft-tissue work by a physical therapist is contraindicated in the left upper abdominal quadrant.[65]

Colon Cancer

Colon cancer is the most frequently diagnosed cancer in the United States, affecting 5–6% of the population.[51,65] These patients may have symptoms that mimic mechanical dysfunction secondary to metastatic presentation in the thoracic spine or rib cage.[65] Risk factors for colon cancer are as follows:

1. Age older than 40 years
2. A history of inflammatory bowel disease
3. Prior cancer
4. Benign colon polyps[65]

The clinician should ask specific questions pertaining to changes in bowel function to screen for cancer symptoms. Nonspecific symptoms of any cancer include malaise, weakness, anorexia, and weight loss.[51,65] Because colon cancer frequently metastasizes to bone, the clinician should be aware of low back symptoms that do not respond to treatment even though provocative testing for lumbar motion segment or sacroiliac joint involvement may have produced positive results.[51]

Aortic Aneurysms

An aortic aneurysm occurs when there is a widening of all three layers (intima, media, and adventitia) of the aorta.[68] It is typically caused by atherosclerosis, a genetically weakened media, trauma, or infection. Three-fourths of aortic aneurysms occur in the abdominal aorta just below the renal arteries.[57] Males older than age 60 years who smoke and are hypertensive are high-risk candidates for developing aneurysms. Aneurysms in the abdominal region may cause severe pain at the thoracolumbar junction.[51] The pain is usually described as a "hot, throbbing" sensation that increases in intensity with physical activity.[68] The patient may also sense a "heartbeat" when supine. The abdominal aorta can be assessed for enlargement through palpation.[51] Acute rupture of an aneurysm causes excruciating pain with hypotension and shock. This is a medical emergency and immediate action must be taken.[68]

Cancer

Primary Skeletal Neoplasm

Neoplasm is any new and abnormal formation of cells that must be considered in a differential musculoskeletal diagnosis. Benign bone lesions occur more frequently than malignant neoplasms. Destruction of the bone in weight-bearing areas may cause weakening and subsequent pathologic fractures.[69] The clinician should be suspicious of pain that is inconsistent with the nature of onset, whether injury or trauma. Osteoblastoma is characteristically found in the spine (34%) and frequently involves the posterior elements. These patients are typically 10–30 years of age, and one-half will present with positive neurologic symptoms.[70] The characteristics of both benign and malignant bone tumors are compared in Table 2-10.[69]

Multiple Myeloma

Myeloma is "a neoplastic proliferation of plasma cells in the bone marrow."[69] Plasma cell myeloma is the most common primary malignant neoplasm of bone. The peak incidence is in males older than age 60 years, with primary sites occurring in the spine, pelvis, and skull.[69] Clinical findings may include pain, bone tenderness, weight loss, and anemia. Pain is described as "deep" and may increase with activity and movement as contrasted with the night pain seen in metastatic cancer. The lesion is frequently located in the spine with low back or rib pain as a chief complaint. Vertebral lesions may lead to pathologic fractures or compression of the cauda equina, causing radicular symptoms.[51,69] An important diagnostic test is to percuss with a reflex hammer over the individual spinous processes to check for symptoms secondary to a pathologic fracture. This test will produce negative findings in a patient with a disc herniation.[67]

Metastatic Cancer

Skeletal metastases occur most commonly from prostate, breast, lung, thyroid, and kidney carcinomas.[51,69] The vascular system is of primary importance in the spread of cancer to secondary sites in bones that have the highest amounts of bone marrow. The most common sites are the pelvis, vertebrae, and proximal portions of the humerus or femur. The most common primary lesion that metastasizes to bone is breast cancer, the frequent site being the thoracic and lumbar vertebral bodies. Forty percent to 50% of prostate and kidney carcinomas will metastasize to bone, usually the pelvis, lumbar vertebrae, and proximal femur. Metastases to the skeletal system occur in the early stages of lung cancer, making treatment difficult. Metastases for carcinoma of the thyroid are found in the skull, ribs, sternum, and spine. The "red flag" symptom of skeletal metastases is severe, constant pain, often at night.[69]

References

1. Naylor A. Intervertebral disc prolapse and degeneration. Spine 1976;1:108.
2. Adams P, Eyre DR, Meir H. Biomechanical aspects of development and ageing of human lumbar intcrvertebral discs. Rheum Rehabil 1977; 16:22.
3. Ham AW, Cormack DH. Histology (8th ed). Philadelphia: Lippincott, 1979;477.
4. Galante J. Tensile properties of the human lumbar annulus fibrosis. Acta Orthop Scand 1967;100[Suppl]:5.
5. Berkson MH. Mechanical properties of the human lumbar spine flexibilities, intradiscal pressures, posterior element influences. Proc Inst Med Chic 1977;31:138.
6. Farfan HF, Cassette JW, Robertson GH, et al. The effects of torsion on the lumbar intervertebral joints: the role of torsion in production of disc degeneration. J Bone Joint Surg 1970;52:468.
7. Twomey LT, Taylor JR. Age changes in lumbar intervertebral discs. Acta Orthop Scand 1986;56:496.
8. Brown T, Hansen RJ, Yerra AJ. Some mechanical tests on the lumbosacral spine with particular reference to the intervertebral discs. J Bone Joint Surg 1957;39:1135.
9. Hirsch C, Nachemson AL. New observations on the mechanical behavior of lumbar discs. Acta Orthop Scand 1954;23:254.
10. Gertzbein SD, Seligman J, Holtby R. Centrode patterns and segmental instability in degenerative disc disease. Spine 1985;10:257.
11. Paris SV. Physical signs of instability. Spine 1985;10:277.
12. McNab I. The traction spur: an indication of segmental instability. J Bone Joint Surg 1971;53:663.
13. Dupuis PR, Yong-Hing K, Cassidy JD, et al. Radiologic diagnosis of degenerative lumbar spinal instability. Spine 1985;10:262.
14. Kirkaldy-Willis WH, Farfan HF. Instability of the lumbar spine. Clin Orthop 1982;165:110.
15. Frymoyer JW, Pope MH, Clements JH, et al. Risk factors in low-back pain: an epidemiological survey. J Bone Joint Surg 1983;65:213.
16. Kellgren JH, Lawrence JS. Osteoarthritis and disk degeneration in an urban population. Ann Rheum Dis 1958;17:388.
17. Wiesel SW, Feffer HL, Rothman RH, et al. Industrial low back pain: a prospective evaluation of a standardized diagnostic and treatment protocol. Spine 1984;9:199.
18. Brant-Zawadzki M, Jensen M. Imaging corner spinal nomenclature. Spine 1995;20:388.
19. Cailliet R. Low Back Syndrome (4th ed). Philadelphia: FA Davis, 1988;275.

20. Ramani PS, Perry RH, Tomlinson BE. Role of the ligamentum flavum in the symptomatology of prolapsed lumbar intervertebral discs. J Neurol Neurosurg Psychiatry 1975;38:550.
21. Yong-Hing K, Reilly J, Kirkaldy-Willis WH. The ligamentum flavum. Spine 1976;1:226.
22. Vernon-Roberts B, Pirie CJ. Degenerative changes in the intervertebral discs of the lumbar spine and their sequelae. Rheum Rehabil 1977;16:13.
23. Lewin T. Osteoarthritis in lumbar synovial joints: a morphological study. Acta Orthop Scand 1964;73[Suppl].
24. Twomey LT, Taylor JR. Physical Therapy of the Low Back. New York: Churchill Livingstone, 1987;2.
25. Tanz SS. Motion of the lumbar spine: a roentgenologic study. AJR Am J Roentgenol 1953;69:399.
26. Penttinen E, Airaksinen O, Pohjolainen O, et al. Subjective relief of back pain at work and patient compliance in corset treatment for degenerative lumbar instability. J Manual Med 1990;5:166.
27. Sashin D. A critical analysis of the anatomy and pathological changes of the sacroiliac joints. J Bone Joint Surg 1930;12:891.
28. McKenzie RA. Mechanical Diagnosis and Therapy for Low Back Pain: Toward a Better Understanding. In LT Twomey, JR Taylor (eds), Physical Therapy of the Low Back. New York: Churchill Livingstone, 1987;159.
29. Schwarzer AC, Aprill CN, Bogduk N. The sacroiliac joint in chronic low back pain. Spine 1995;20:31.
30. Potter N, Rothstein J. Intertester reliability for selected clinical test of the sacroiliac joint. J Phys Ther 1985;65:1671.
31. Lauerman WC, Caine JE. Isthmic spondylolisthesis in the adult. J Am Acad Orthop Surg 1996;12:201.
32. Wiltse LL, Newman PH, McNab I. Classification of spondylolysis and spondylolisthesis. Clin Orthop 1976;117:23.
33. Magora A, Schwartz A. Relation between the low back pain syndrome and x-ray findings: lysis and olisthesis. Scand J Rehabil Med 1980;12:47.
34. Commandre FA, Taillan B, Gagnerie F, et al. Spondylolysis and spondylolisthesis in young athletes: 28 cases. J Sports Med 1988;28:104.
35. Frederickson BE, Baker D, McHolick WJ, et al. The natural history of spondylolysis and spondylolisthesis. J Bone Joint Surg 1984;66:699.
36. Friberg O. Lumbar instability: a dynamic approach by traction-compression radiography. Spine 1987;12:119.
37. Virta L, Rönnemaa T. The association of mild-moderate isthmic lumbar spondylolisthesis and low back pain in middle-aged patients is weak and it only occurs in women. Spine 1993;18:1496.
38. Sato H, Kikuchi S. The natural history of radiographic instability of the lumbar spine. Spine 1993;18:2075.

39. Magora A, Schwartz A. Relation between the low back pain syndrome and x-ray findings: spina bifida occulta. Scand J Rehabil Med 1980;12:9.

40. Weinstein SL, Zavala DC, Ponseti IV, et al. Idiopathic scoliosis: long-term follow-up and prognosis in untreated patients. J Bone Joint Surg 1981;63:702.

41. Connolly PJ, Von Schroeder PV, Johnson GE, et al. Adolescent idiopathic scoliosis: long-term effect of instrumentation extending to the lumbar spine. J Bone Joint Surg 1995;77:1210.

42. Grieve GP. Bony and Soft-Tissue Anomalies of the Vertebral Column. In GP Grieve (ed), Modern Manual Therapy of the Vertebral Column. Edinburgh: Churchill Livingstone, 1986;3.

43. Farfan HF, Sullivan JD. The relation of facet orientation to intervertebral disc failure. Can J Surg 1967;10:179.

44. Vanharanta H, Floyd T, Ohnmeiss DD, et al. The relationship of facet tropism to degenerative disc disease. Spine 1993;18:1000.

45. Frymoyer JW, Andersson GBJ. Clinical Classification. In MH Pope, GBJ Andersson, JW Frymoyer (eds), Occupational Low Back Pain: Assessment, Treatment, and Prevention. St. Louis: Mosby–Year Book, 1991;58.

46. Amundsen T, Weber H, Lilleas F, et al. Lumbar spinal stenosis: clinical and radiologic features. Spine 1995;20:1178.

47. White AH, Anderson R. Conservative Care of Low Back Pain. Baltimore: Williams & Wilkins, 1991;225.

48. Turek S. Orthopaedics: Principles and Their Applications. Philadelphia: Lippincott, 1977;387.

49. Berkow R (ed). The Merck Manual of Diagnosis and Therapy. Rahway, NJ: Merck, 1977;815–1335.

50. Kirchner JT. Reiter's syndrome: a possibility in patients with reactive arthritis. Postgrad Med 1995;97:111.

51. Koopmeiners M, Boissonnault WG. Medical Diagnostics for the Physical Therapist. Presented at the Institute of Graduate Physical Therapy course; January 15–17, 1993; Washington, DC.

52. Borenstein D. Prevalence and treatment outcome of primary and secondary fibromyalgia in patients with spinal pain. Spine 1995;20:796.

53. Caldron PH. Screening for Rheumatic Disease. In WG Boissonnault (ed), Examination in Physical Therapy Practice: Screening for Medical Disease. New York: Churchill Livingstone, 1991;237.

54. Lander P, Hadjipavlou A. Intradiscal invasion of Paget's disease of the spine. Spine 1991;16:46.

55. Ling FW, King PM, Myers CA. Screening for Female Urogenital System Disease. In WG Boissonnault (ed), Examination in Physical Therapy Practice: Screening for Medical Disease. New York: Churchill Livingstone, 1991;124.

56. Goodman C, Snyder T. Differential Diagnosis in Physical Therapy: Musculoskeletal and Systemic Conditions. Philadelphia: Saunders, 1990;344.
57. Thorn G (ed). Harrison's Principles of Internal Medicine (8th ed). New York: McGraw-Hill, 1977.
58. Tanagho EA, McAninch JW. Smith's General Urology (12th ed). Norwalk, CT: Appleton & Lange, 1984;220–295.
59. Porterfield JA, DeRosa C. Mechanical Low Back Pain: Perspectives in Functional Anatomy. Philadelphia: Saunders, 1991;169–186.
60. Fast A, Shapiro D, Ducommun EJ, et al. Low-back pain in pregnancy. Spine 1987;12:368.
61. Fair WR, Fuks ZY, Scher HI. Cancer of the Urethra and Penis. In VT Devita, S Hellman, SA Rosenberg (eds), Cancer: Principles and Practice of Oncology (4th ed). Philadelphia: Lippincott, 1993;1116.
62. McLinn DM, Boissonnault WG. Screening for Male Urogenital System Disease. In WG Boissonnault (ed), Examination in Physical Therapy Practice: Screening for Medical Disease. New York: Churchill Livingstone, 1991;121.
63. Fair WR, Fuks ZY, Scher HI, et al. Cancer of the Bladder. In VT Devita, S Hellman, SA Rosenberg (eds), Cancer: Principles and Practice of Oncology (4th ed). Philadelphia: Lippincott, 1993;1054.
64. Moul JW. Prostatitis: sorting out the different causes. Postgrad Med 1993;94:191.
65. Koopmeiners MB. Screening for Gastrointestinal System Disease. In WG Boissonnault (ed), Examination in Physical Therapy Practice: Screening for Medical Disease. NewYork: Churchill Livingstone, 1991;105.
66. Williams PL, Warwick R. Gray's Anatomy (35th British ed). Philadelphia: Saunders, 1973;1288.
67. Boissonnault WG, Janos SC. Screening for Medical Disease: Physical Therapy Assessment and Treatment Principles. In WG Boissonnault (ed), Examination in Physical Therapy Practice: Screening for Medical Disease. New York: Churchill Livingstone, 1991;1.
68. Michel TH, Downing J. Screening for Cardiovascular System Disease. In WG Boissonnault (ed), Examination in Physical Therapy Practice: Screening for Medical Disease. New York: Churchill Livingstone, 1991;33.
69. Randall T, McMahon K. Screening for Musculoskeletal System Disease. In WG Boissonnault (ed), Examination in Physical Therapy Practice: Screening for Medical Disease. New York: Churchill Livingstone, 1991;199.
70. Healy JH, Ghelman B. Osteoid osteoma and osteoblastoma: ten most common bone and joint tumors. Clin Orthop 1986;204:76.

II

Evaluation

3

Patient History: Diagnostic and Clinical Significance

Brian P. D'Orazio and
Cynthia Burks Starling

The examination of a patient begins by taking a thorough history. This process is initiated by the patient's filling out a history form with information specific to his or her complaint, along with a general medical history. Information obtained from a thorough history often provides the key to a patient's problem. Expert clinicians begin the process of developing a working diagnosis by interpreting the patient's written history before directly communicating with the patient.[1] In the appendix to this chapter is a logically arranged history form that becomes part of the patient's medical record and should be readily accessible for future reference (Appendix 3-1).

Well-trained support personnel can preliminarily confirm the patient's history and brief the clinician. The clinician begins by first identifying areas in the patient's written history that are incomplete or that require further clarification. The entire process assists in developing a working diagnosis, in directing the physical examination, and in establishing both the patient's and the clinician's treatment goals. The remainder of this chapter examines how to obtain a history that assists in formulating a working diagnosis.

Initial Information Gathering

Most histories begin by obtaining general patient information (see Appendix 3-1). The reason for most of this information is obvious, but a few points deserve elaboration.

Other than for record keeping, the patient's name may indicate an ethnic background or race that predisposes the patient to certain medical conditions. Although studies vary regarding differences in pain threshold among different ethnic groups, there is better agreement in the literature regarding differences in the expression or reporting of pain as well as in preference of treatment method. Clark[2] summarized the ethnic and cultural differences of patients as follows: "[P]robably all of the differences in pain thresholds reported among various ethnocultural and religious groups are due to cultural differences in the criterion for reporting pain and not to differences in the sensory experience of pain itself." The author cites studies that Anglo-Americans generally prefer pills or injections for pain relief, whereas Chinese patients prefer external agents such as salves, compresses, or massage.[2]

The patient's age should be considered in relationship to typical age-related diseases. A history of insidious low back pain (LBP) at age 60 years, in combination with other findings, could suggest spinal stenosis, arthritic changes, or, for men, prostate cancer.

The patient's occupation offers information about physical activity level. Specific types of back problems are more likely to occur in patients with sedentary jobs or among patients who commute great distances, than in patients who have heavy manual labor jobs.

Information on the number and ages of children provides clues about the patient's lifestyle, including child care activities, which could predispose the patient to back strains. For women, the number and types of births may indicate the likelihood of abdominal muscle insufficiency, especially if any of the deliveries were by cesarean section. The number of pregnancies should also be investigated, since multiple miscarriages may indicate gynecologic problems that could be related to the patient's LBP.

The names of all health care practitioners consulted for this condition should be provided by the patient. Treatment by multiple practitioners does not necessarily indicate that all physiologic complaints have been thoroughly investigated. It is reasonable to assume, however, that patients who have seen multiple practitioners have not found a satisfactory explanation for their problem and have not received successful treatment.

Sleep History

Often overlooked is the average number of hours the patient sleeps each night. Patients who consistently received 4 or fewer hours of sleep per night need to have this problem thoroughly explored. Reduced sleep is associated with many conditions and is a common indicator of depression, anxiety, or stress. Any of these conditions can be a barrier to recovery. The perpetuation of pain and even the production of pain can have its basis in depression, a subject that is discussed later in this chapter and also in Chapter 5. Other conditions associated with lack of sleep include rhabdomyalgia, hormonal imbalances, sleep disorders, cancer, and vascular disorders. Occasionally, patients will indicate that 4 hours of sleep or less is normal. This response should be viewed cautiously, as it generally indicates a very unhealthy lifestyle, unrecognized depression, or other issues that the patient has not discussed. Practically speaking, 4 hours of sleep does not give the patient's mind and body enough rest to either manage his or her symptoms or participate in an extensive exercise program.

Eating Patterns

Recent changes in eating patterns may indicate several disease processes, including depression. If the patient indicates he or she is eating a normal amount but losing weight, further medical investigation should be pursued to rule out cancer or other serious medical problems. If the patient's appetite has been reduced, clinical depression should be suspected, although pain and restricted activity may also cause a reduced appetite.

Bowel and Bladder Habits

If recent changes in bowel or bladder habits have not been thoroughly investigated and did not have an obvious cause, the questionnaires in Appendixes 3-2, 3-3, and 3-4 can be used as a screening mechanism to assist in identifying potential pathologic conditions that should be referred to a physician for further investigation. For example, if urinary frequency has increased, this could indicate a urogenital infection. Patients with abdominal or iliopsoas muscle involvement, however, sometimes describe a sense of increased frequency and urgency in the absence of positive tests for infection. A loss of bladder control may indicate a sacral plexus injury from a significant disc herniation, which requires immediate surgical attention. This is also true for loss of bowel control. A decrease in bowel activity is associated with constipation, diverticulosis, cancer, and other gastrointestinal disorders. People in the active stages of diverticulitis or who have Crohn's disease often have associated LBP.

Medical History

Appendix 3-1 includes a brief medical and psychosocial history. Each one of these variables may have significant consequences regarding treatment and the patient's ability to recover from the current condition. Only a few of these conditions are discussed in this section of the chapter.

Diabetes

A history of diabetes can indicate a poor prognosis for recovery, especially if the diabetes is not well controlled. Patients with diabetes, even those who are diligent about monitoring blood and urine levels, often recover more slowly than other patients. Diabetic neuropathies can mimic nerve root involvement and need to be considered in the differential diagnosis. Furthermore, in patients with advanced diabetic conditions, general neuropathies can create muscular weakness, leading to pain associated with the normal activities of daily living. Diabetes has also been cited as a source of sciatica.[3]

Cancer

A history of cancer must be thoroughly investigated. Even when the patient has undergone testing for additional cancers, the physical examination and history should be closely correlated. Cancer of the gastrointestinal tract, in particular, is associated with LBP and pelvic girdle pain. Fever, chills, and sweats may indicate many conditions, ranging from cancer to menopause. If these conditions are associated with unexplained weight change, cancer should be strongly suspected.

Depression

Depression is a category that many patients often do not recognize or will not acknowledge. If this category is left unanswered, the clinician should question the patient about a past or present history of depression. Situational depressions often arise as the result of LBP and its attendant disability. Once the patient's condition begins responding to treatment, the depression commonly resolves. If the depression does not abate or if the patient's disability is going to be protracted, consultation with mental health care providers should be considered. Tests for depression that are nonthreatening to the patient and quickly administered and scored by the clinician are discussed later in the chapter.

Substance Abuse and Sexual Difficulty

The two most underreported categories in the personal medical history are substance abuse and sexual difficulty. Often the patient will answer negatively to experiencing sexual difficulty associated with LBP and yet the patient's physical examination clearly demonstrates a severe movement dysfunction. This discrepancy between the patient's report of experiencing sexual difficulty and the clinician's examination of the patient's impairments and disabilities should be investigated. The most common reason for underreporting sexual difficulty is embarrassment; however, other factors may include depression, an inability to engage in sexual activity because of other medical conditions, or abstinence. This area should be thoroughly investigated for many reasons, including the possibility that the patient is exacerbating symptoms through sexual intercourse or that the symptoms present have been caused by sexual intercourse.

Patients with a history of substance abuse who are recovering—alcoholics or addicts—typically respond affirmatively on the history form. The more difficult patient is the one who has become dependent on alcohol or drugs in an effort to manage symptoms. These patients will generally answer negatively on the history form. Not only is substance abuse a barrier to recovery and one that may exacerbate depression, it is a also safety concern in the clinic. If the physical therapist's observations lead him or her to suspect substance abuse and the interview confirms these suspicions, it is important that the physical therapist discuss this with the patient and organize a plan of action to remove this barrier.

Contributing Factors

Appendix 3-1 also lists potential contributing variables that may be germane to the patient's current complaints of LBP. The first problem, injury, may include an injury unrelated specifically to the lumbar spine. As an example, the patient may have sustained a knee injury that he or she did not think was associated with the LBP. The patient's gait, however, may have been altered and this abnormality may be relevant.

Being overtired before an injury could signify a reason for the injury to occur or may indicate the patient's workload was too great for his or her strength and endurance. It is not unusual in factories to see injuries occurring near the end of shifts because of muscular fatigue.

Sustained postures or heavy lifting are obvious in their implications regarding the patient's LBP. This list of contributing factors may help the patient think of predisposing variables possibly related to the current chief complaint.

Medical Testing

The section of Appendix 3-1 titled "Medical Testing" lists commonly performed tests related to LBP. The patient's interpretation of the medical tests should never be regarded as a substitute for independent confirmation through appropriate medical personnel, especially when test results are critical to treatment. Often, patients do not understand some of the medical terminology or are not sure which test was performed; therefore, the clinician should ask appropriate questions to ensure the patient understands the tests listed.

Symptoms

In the symptom section of the history form, the patient is asked to describe his or her chief complaint (see Appendix 3-1). When verbally confirming the patient's history, the clinician may need to ask the patient to rate multiple complaints in order of severity if more than one complaint is listed. In the case of multiple pain sources, separate pain scales need to be used.

Nature of Symptoms

The nature of the patient's symptoms should involve a list of questions that helps the clinician understand how and when the symptoms began, what specific activity or pathologic condition is relevant to the patient's chief complaint, and how the patient experiences the pain. Under the section of the history form titled "Description of Discomfort," the specific descriptors are often not as important as the number of items checked. If the patient is checking many items, the clinician should be sensitive to the possibility that symptom magnification may be an issue. Sensations such as burning and cramping may indicate vascular or neurologic problems. Certainly, tingling and numbness can be signs of neurologic involvement; however, patients often confuse numbness with tingling. This should be confirmed verbally with the patient during the physical examination.

Pain Behavior

The next section of the history form is related to symptoms and their behavior. Pain can be constant, intermittent, or a combination of both. If intermittent, pain frequency communicates information about the degree of disability and the irritability of the problem. This also provides the clinician with a criterion by which to measure change after treatment is initiated. In patients with intermittent pain, it is important to assess the length of time that the symptoms last. In patients whose symptoms are constant, normal musculoskeletal symptoms have diurnal variations, some of which occur as the result of changes in activity. Even in chronic conditions, most patients learn to manage the problem in such a way that symptoms are minimized for at least part of the day. If there appear to be no diurnal variations in the patient's complaint, other medical conditions such as cancer should be suspected. This is especially true if the patient tends to have more nighttime pain. The lack of diurnal variations may also indicate symptom magnification syndrome (SMS).

Diurnal variations in symptoms can be related to other pathologic conditions. Pain from conditions that involve an inflammatory response, such as connective tissue diseases, is typically characterized as varying in intensity, with increased discomfort when arising and decreased discomfort after moving around. The patient may also describe more discomfort when sleeping or an inability to sleep as long because of pain. Inflammation of any tissue can create this type of response. Inflammatory changes can be self-perpetuating, leading to chronic pain.

In contrast, a patient who arises with little or no pain and then experiences progressive symptoms through the day may be describing a fatigue-related response. This can be secondary to inadequate trunk endurance, postural deviations placing abnormal stresses on musculoskeletal structures, diminished force production, or a psychosocial dysfunction.

Often, patients are unable to describe diurnal variations in their pain. Directing the patient to describe his or her symptoms with specific activities throughout the day may be helpful. It is not uncommon, however, for the pain intensity to be so great that essentially the patient cannot distinguish which specific activities exacerbate symptoms.

Specific activities that exacerbate symptoms may be of diagnostic significance. For example, pain that increases with walking and is reduced when the patient is bent slightly forward may suggest spinal stenosis. Most patients with a lumbar disc herniation report that sitting and standing are poorly tolerated while climbing the stairs may be fairly comfortable. Furthermore, most patients are able to find positions that reduce their symptoms and this information is also helpful.

Pain experienced in the low back or into the lower extremities when coughing or sneezing is attributable to many problems; however, disc disease must be ruled out. Typically, patients with disc herniations will protect their backs by flexing one or both hips when they cough or sneeze and try to avoid coughing and sneezing altogether.

Location of Symptoms

The nature of the patient's chief complaint can be described further through the use of pain diagrams. Pain diagrams should show all quadrants of the body. A key allows the patient to more precisely express the nature of the pain.

Psychological dysfunctions such as depression, anxiety, hypochondriasis, and hysteria are measurable by personality inventories. Anatomically implausible distributions of pain noted in drawings and abnormal pain behaviors during physical examination also suggest psychological dysfunctions.[4–6] Southwick and White recommended a battery of the following tests for identifying psychological problems: the Minnesota Multiphasic Personality Inventory (MMPI), the Middlesex Hospital Questionnaire, and the Pain Drawing diagram.[7] Flores and colleagues reported that the Pain Drawing offers an assessment of pain location, severity, and anxiety or somatization, thereby having both psychological and anatomic components.[8] As a diagnostic tool it is inexpensive, easily completed by the patient, and gives the clinician an immediate overview of the pain's location. Ohnmeiss and colleagues reported that a literature review reveals pain drawings should be used as an initial screening tool, along with several other tests, and has limited prognostic capabilities when used alone.[9]

Other

The section of the history form titled "Other" is the final part of the patient's history. This section allows for communication of anything else the patient feels he or she had not previously been able to communicate. Most of the time, all relevant information has been gathered. The patient's report of previous treatment outcomes is important. Treatment programs that appear to be appropriate and yet have been unsuccessful may alert the clinician to the possibility that unrecognized barriers to recovery exist.

Finally, the patient's goals should be established. The history form is the beginning of the patient establishing goals for treatment and can be the beginning of the clinician establishing goals for discharge. Clinicians should empower the patient to manage his or her symptoms, accomplish activities of daily living, and return to hobbies and employment. If a patient cannot think of any goals, the physical therapist should ask what activity the patient misses the most that he or she was able to do before the injury.

Pain Behavior Assessment

In many circumstances, further information needs to be obtained from the patient to assess the influence of multiple factors on the patient's disability and how that disability compares to the patient's impairment. The simplest definition of disability is what the patient believes he or she can do, whereas impairment defines the objective limits of strength, endurance, range of motion, coordination, and balance. Under ideal conditions, the physical impairment matches the patient's disability. When a substantial disparity between impairment and disability exists, additional testing needs to be performed.

The role of psychosocial variables in chronic LBP is well published. The clinician has the responsibility of recognizing and investigating how emotions may be affecting the patient's physiologic function. Flores and colleagues described the "recent trend in the use of objective quantifiable instruments encompassing the physical, psychological, and socioeconomic parameters of outcomes research in painful disorders."[8] Psychological tests can provide needed information to help the clinician confirm or deny other clinical findings and should be a part of the patient history.[10] No single psychological instrument can measure pain, predict success or evaluate changes in improvement or function. However, if these tests are used as supplementary findings, they are invaluable tools in corroborating the clinician's findings.[10]

Screening for Depression

The MMPI is widely recognized as the most standardized, objective psychological instrument.[10] It is a 567-item test of true-and-false questions. Standard scales measure the test validity and various psychological issues, particularly symptom magnification. This is a lengthy test and potentially threatening to patients because of the sensitive nature of some questions, and is not used in our clinic for these reasons. The Millon Behavioral Health Inventory (MBHI) is similar to the MMPI, but much shorter, with only 150 true-and-false questions. This test provides useful information on coping styles and psychopathology,[8] and is successful in predicting the physical functioning of LBP patients.[10,11]

We have found the Beck Depression Inventory (BDI), which is included in Matheson's Behavioral Medicine Profile (Appendix 3-5), to be an excellent tool for evaluating depression and the most expedient way to identify suicidal ideation. Twenty-one multiple-choice questions are posed with directions for the patient to circle the response that most nearly reflects the way he or she has been feeling the last several days.[12] Kendall and colleagues recommended a multiple method assessment, including the structured clinical interview and repeated testings.[13]

Assessments of Pain and Function

We have found the following instruments, in addition to the BDI, to be good self-report measures in establishing a LBP patient's psychological profile: The Oswestry Low Back Pain Disability Questionnaire, the McGill Pain Questionnaire (MPQ), and the three 10-cm pain scales.

Oswestry Low Back Pain Disability Questionnaire

The Oswestry questionnaire is designed to elicit, from its multiple choice format, how LBP has affected the patient's life[14] (Appendix 3-6). This is an excellent means of determining, on the first visit, how the patient perceives his or her level of function. With the questionnaire repeated periodically during treatment, it is hoped that the physical therapist will witness an improvement in the patient's score corresponding to an improvement in the patient's functional level.

McGill Pain Questionnaire

The McGill Pain Questionnaire (MPQ) (Appendix 3-7) consists of 78 adjectives divided into three categories—sensory-discriminative, affective, and evaluative—that Melzack theorizes correlate with the three categories of pain.[15] The patient is asked to check adjectives from the questionnaire that best describe his or her pain. This test is useful when administered at the beginning and end of their referral to document any changes in their perception of pain that might be related to treatment.[16]

Pain Scales

The Pain Scales consist of three horizontal 10-cm lines[17] (Figure 3-1). One line is used to rate pain "at its least," one for pain "at its worst," and one for pain "now." The left side of each line is marked as "no pain" and the right side is marked "maximum pain." The patient uses a vertical line on each of the horizontal scales to indicate the pain level in each circumstance. Figure 3-1 shows the typical responses of symptom magnifiers (SM) and normal persons (N).

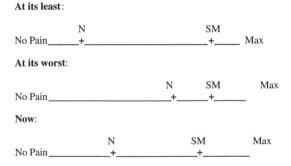

Indicate on the pain scale below by making a line where your pain is at its least, where it is at its worst, and where it is now:

At its least:

At its worst:

Now:

Figure 3-1 The Pain Scales. (N = normal [marks made left of midline]; SM = symptom magnification [marks made at or to the right of midline].) (Reproduced with permission from RB King. Managing Symptom Magnification. In BP D'Orazio [ed], Back Pain Rehabilitation. Boston: Andover Medical Publishers, 1993;132.)

Roland and Morris Disability Questionnaire

Functional status can also be measured by use of the Roland and Morris Disability Questionnaire (RMQ), which is an abbreviated version of the Sickness Impact Profile (SIP)[18] (Appendix 3-8). The RMQ contains 24 items of the SIP that describe various activities of daily living. Stratford and colleagues described this instrument as one that can be self-administered and completed in 5 minutes.[16] An item is scored 0 if it is not thought to be applicable by the respondent, and receives a 1 if it is applicable. In scoring, the total may range from 0 for no disability to 24 for severe disability. Deyo found good reliability ratings and moderate validity ratings in both the RMQ and SIP.[19]

Conclusion

The process of examining the patient's written and verbal history may leave a lasting impression on the patient. Allowing the patient to adequately vocalize his or her complaint is extremely important in developing patient rapport. Although patients should be directed in their comments so as not to waste time on irrelevant issues, the combination of a thorough written history and verbal confirmation demonstrates the clinician's commitment to the patient.

The patient's history provides us with a wealth of knowledge that helps establish a diagnosis. The process of developing a diagnosis is analogous to solving a puzzle. The picture that emerges becomes clearer as we obtain more pieces. The patient history provides many pieces to the puzzle, and its importance cannot be overstated.

References

1. Payton OD. Clinical reasoning process in physical therapy. Phys Ther 1985;65:924.
2. Clark WC. Pain and Suffering. In JA Downey, SJ Myers, EG Gonzalez, JS Leiberman (eds), The Physiological Basis of Rehabilitation Medicine (2nd ed). Boston: Butterworth–Heinemann, 1994;705.
3. Naftulin S, Fast A, Thomas M. Diabetic lumbar radiculopathy: sciatica without disc herniation. Spine 1993;18:2419.
4. Andersson GBJ, Svensson HO, Oden A. The intensity of work recovery in low back pain. Spine 1983;8:880.
5. Frymoyer JW, Rosen JC, Clements J, Pope MH. Psychologic factors in low-back-pain disability. Clin Orthop 1985;195:178.
6. Ransford AO, Cairns D, Mooney V. The pain drawing as an aid to the psychologic evaluation of patients with low-back pain. Spine 1976;1:127.

7. Southwick SM, White AA. Current concepts review: the use of psychological tests in the evaluation of low back pain. J Bone Joint Surg 1983;65A:560.
8. Flores L, Gatchel RJ, Polatin PB. Objectification of functional improvement after nonoperative care. Spine 1997;22:1622.
9. Ohnmeiss DD, Vanharanta H, Guyer RD. The association between pain drawings and computed tomographic/discographic pain responses. Spine 1995;20:729.
10. Drukteinis AM, Slovenko R (eds). The Psychology of Back Pain: A Clinical and Legal Handbook. Springfield, IL: Charles C Thomas, 1996;62.
11. Gatchel RJ, Mayer TG, Capra P, et al. Millon Behavioral Health Inventory: its utility in predicting physical function in patients with low-back pain. Arch Phys Med Rehabil 1986;67:878.
12. Matheson LN. Symptom Magnification Syndrome: Behavioral Medicinal Profile. Presented at the Roy Matheson and Associates Work and Assessment Systems Workshop, May 28–31, 1992, Pittsburgh, PA.
13. Kendell PC, Hollon SD, Beck AT, Hammen CL, et al. Issues and recommendations regarding use of the Beck Depression Inventory. Cognitive Therapy and Research 1987;11:289.
14. Fairbank JCT, Couper J, Davies JB, O'Brien JP. The Oswestery low back pain disability questionnaire. Physiotherapy 1980;66:271.
15. Melzack R. The McGill Pain Questionnaire: major properties and scoring methods. Pain 1975;1:277.
16. Stratford PW, Binkley J, Soloman P, et al. Assessing change over time in patients with low back pain. Phys Ther 1994;74:528.
17. King RB. Managing Symptom Magnification. In BP D'Orazio (ed), Back Pain Rehabilitation. Boston: Andover Medical Publishers, 1993;132.
18. Roland M, Morris R. A study of the natural history of back pain, part I: development of a reliable and sensitive measure of disability in low-back pain. Spine 1983;8:141.
19. Deyo RA, Diehl AK. Measuring physical and psychosocial function in patients with low-back pain. Spine 1983;8:635.

Chapter 3
Appendixes

Appendix 3-1

**Orthopedic and Sports
Physical Therapy Associates, Inc.**
312 Butler Road, 421 Chatham Square Office Park
Fredericksburg, Virginia 22405
(540) 373-3031

General patient information

Today's date_____

Name _____ Date of birth _____ Age _____

Sex _____ Occupation _____ No. of children _____

No. of pregnancies _____ Height _____ Weight _____

Name of referring physician _____

Date of most recent examination _____

Date of next appointment _____

Please list names of physicians, therapists, or other practitioners previously seen for this condition. _____

_____

Please list all current medications (also include nonprescription medications).

_____

Please list all previous prescription medications.

_____

Average no. of hours of sleep per night _____ Is this normal for you? _____

Have you experienced any recent changes in eating patterns? Yes/No

If yes, please explain _____

Have you experienced any recent changes in bowel or bladder habits? Yes/No

If yes, please explain _____

Medical history

Personal history of	Please circle one of the following:	Please include additional information for clarification.
1. Heart disease	Yes/No	_____
2. Stroke	Yes/No	_____
3. Respiratory problems	Yes/No	_____
4. Diabetes	Yes/No	_____
5. Arthritis	Yes/No	_____
6. Cancer	Yes/No	_____
7. Allergies	Yes/No	_____
8. High blood pressure	Yes/No	_____
9. Fever/chills/sweats	Yes/No	_____
10. Unexplained weight change	Yes/No	_____
11. Depression	Yes/No	_____
12. Nausea/vomiting	Yes/No	_____
13. Numbness	Yes/No	_____
14. Weakness	Yes/No	_____
15. Fainting	Yes/No	_____

16. Dizziness	Yes/No	_____
17. Night pain	Yes/No	_____
18. Shortness of breath	Yes/No	_____
19. Sexual difficulty	Yes/No	_____
20. Smoking	Yes/No	_____
21. Mental illness/ psychological consultation	Yes/No	_____
22. Substance abuse	Yes/No	_____
23. Family medical problems	Yes/No	
24. Other medical problems, illness, or disease	Yes/No	_____
25. Surgery	Yes/No	_____

If yes, list all prior surgeries and dates _____

_____

_____

Contributing factors

Problems possibly pertinent to your present condition	Please circle one of the following:	Please include additional information for clarification.
1. Injury	Yes/No	_____
2. Illness	Yes/No	_____
3. Virus just prior	Yes/No	_____
4. Flu just prior	Yes/No	_____
5. Overtired just prior	Yes/No	_____
6. Sustained or unusual position	Yes/No	_____
7. Unusual activity	Yes/No	_____
8. Heavy lifting	Yes/No	_____
9. Immobilization (e.g., cast, brace)	Yes/No	_____

Medical testing (special tests pertinent to patient's current problem)

Test	Yes/No	Date	Where performed	Your interpretation of your test results
X-ray	____	____	_____	_____
Blood or urine tests	____	____	_____	_____
Electromyogram	____	____	_____	_____
Computed tomography scan	____	____	_____	_____
Magnetic resonance imaging scan	____	____	_____	_____
Myelogram	____	____	_____	_____
Arthrogram	____	____	_____	_____
Stress test	____	____	_____	_____
Other	____	____	_____	_____

Symptoms

A. Nature of symptoms
  1. Chief complaint: _____
  2. Severity of discomfort at present time (please rate by circling the appropriate number)

  0   1   2   3   4   5   6   7   8   9   10
  No pain   Worst pain you have
                                                 ever experienced in your life

  3. Onset
     a. When did your pain begin? (Please provide date.) _____
     b. Was the onset of your pain sudden _____ gradual ____ other ____?
     c. Where and how did it begin (activity and specific cause)
        _____
        _____

     d. Which of the following describes your problem?
        Worse _____ Better _____ Not changing _____
     e. Just before this onset, were you completely free of discomfort where you have it now? ____
     f. If not, please list the date and cause of injury and duration and treatment of prior episodes. _____
        _____

  4. Description of discomfort
     a. Ache ____ pain ____ other _____
     b. Sharp ____ dull _____ other _____
     c. Paresthesias (strange sensations): pins and needles ____ numbness ____
        tingling ____ burning ____ other ____ none ____
     d. Throbbing ____ cramping ____ other ____
B. Behavior of symptoms
  1. Which of the following describes your discomfort?
     Constant _____ intermittent _____
     a. If intermittent, how often does it recur? _____
     b. When it recurs, how long does it last? _____
     c. How long can you be free of discomfort? _____
  2. Describe your discomfort over a typical day.
     a. On arising: No pain ___ less pain ___ more pain ___ no change ___
     b. As the morning
        progresses: No pain ___ less pain ___ more pain ___ no change ___
     c. Mid-day: No pain ___ less pain ___ more pain ___ no change ___
     d. Before bedtime: No pain ___ less pain ___ more pain ___ no change ___
  3. What activities or positions aggravate your problem? _____
     _____
  4. What activities or positions relieve your problem? _____
     _____
  5. Do you experience discomfort when you cough or sneeze? _____

6. Effect of rest
   a. What is the effect of rest on your discomfort? Relieves _____ makes worse _____ no change _____
   b. Does your discomfort ever wake you at night? _____
   c. If yes, please describe how often, and if you can get back to sleep.
      _____

7. Location
   a. Present: Exactly where is your discomfort? Mark those areas on the body diagram that represent the location of your symptoms. Draw the following symbols onto the body diagrams to indicate the location and intensity of pain or numbness.

      ✔✔✔ Minimal to moderate pain

      ■■■ Severe pain

      →→→ Radiating pain

      ✖✖✖ Numbness

                        Right   Left

   b. Past:
      i. When your problem began, was your discomfort in exactly the same location as you have it now? _____
      ii. If the position of the discomfort has changed, how did the position of the discomfort progress from the original location? _____
         _____

C. Is there anything else pertinent to your problem that hasn't been covered?
   _____
   _____

D. Have you had previous therapy? _____
   1. What was the outcome? _____
      _____
   2. What are your current expectations? _____
      _____
   3. What are your goals? _____
      _____

Appendix 3-2

Female Urogenital System*

Have you noticed or do you have	Please circle one of the following	Please provide additional information that you believe is important to understanding your present condition.
1. Irregularities in your menstrual cycle	Yes/No	_____
2. Vaginal bleeding after menopause	Yes/No	_____
3. Problems with fertility	Yes/No	_____
4. Unusual vaginal discharge	Yes/No	_____
5. Vaginal or associated pain with intercourse	Yes/No	_____
6. History of venereal disease	Yes/No	_____
7. History of bladder or kidney infections	Yes/No	_____
8. An increased frequency of urination	Yes/No	_____
9. An increased sense of urgency with urination	Yes/No	_____
10. Difficulty controlling urination (incontinence)	Yes/No	_____
11. Pain with urination	Yes/No	_____
12. Blood in your urine	Yes/No	_____

---

*Adapted with permission from WG Boissonnault, C Bass. Pathological origins of trunk and neck pain: part I—pelvic and abdominal visceral disorders. J Orthop Sports Phys Ther 1990;12:192.

Appendix 3-3

Male Urogenital System*

Have you noticed or do you have	Please circle one of the following	Please provide additional information that you believe is important to understanding your present condition.
1. Impotence	Yes/No	_____
2. Pain during or immediately after ejaculation	Yes/No	_____
3. Unusual discharge from your penis	Yes/No	_____
4. History of venereal disease	Yes/No	_____
5. History of bladder or kidney infections	Yes/No	_____
6. Diminished flow of urine	Yes/No	_____
7. Increased frequency of urination	Yes/No	_____
8. Increased urgency for urination	Yes/No	_____
9. Difficulty controlling urination (incontinence)	Yes/No	_____
10. Pain with urination	Yes/No	_____
11. Blood in your urine	Yes/No	_____

*Adapted with permission from WG Boissonnault, C Bass. Pathological origins of trunk and neck pain: part I—pelvic and abdominal visceral disorders. J Orthop Sports Phys Ther 1990;12:192.

Appendix 3-4

Gastrointestinal System*

Have you noticed or do you have	Please circle one of the following	Please provide additional information that you believe is important to understanding your present condition.
1. Frequent diarrhea	Yes/No	_____
2. Frequent constipation	Yes/No	_____
3. A change in the color of your stools	Yes/No	_____
4. Bleeding from the rectum	Yes/No	_____
5. Liver or gallbladder disease	Yes/No	_____
6. More of a yellowish skin color than normal	Yes/No	_____
7. Specific foods that are not well tolerated that were tolerated previously	Yes/No	_____
8. Pain or difficulty with swallowing	Yes/No	_____
9. An increase in indigestion, heartburn, or nausea	Yes/No	_____
10. Vomiting not associated with the flu	Yes/No	_____

*Adapted with permission from WG Boissonnault, C Bass. Pathological origins of trunk and neck pain: part I—pelvic and abdominal visceral disorders. J Orthop Sports Phys Ther 1990;12:192.

Appendix 3-5

Behavioral Medicine Profile*

Employment and Rehabilitation Institute of California

Leonard N. Matheson, Ph.D.

Name: _____ **Date:** _____

What are your goals?

Everybody has goals. We are interested in your goals. Please rank the following goals in order of importance. Place a "1" next to the goal that is most important to you, a "4" next to the goal that is least important, and either "2" or "3" next to each of the other goals. There are no right or wrong answers. We really want to find out what is important to you.

_____ To keep working or get back to work.

_____ To get rid of my pain.

_____ To resume activities that are important to me.

_____ To get my pain under control.

How are you doing?

This questionnaire contains groups of statements. Please read each group of statements carefully. Then pick out the one statement in each group that best describes the way you have been doing **during the past week, including today!** Circle the number beside the statement you have chosen. **Be sure to read all the statements in each group before making your choice.**

1. 0......I make decisions about as well as I ever could.
   1.....I put off making decisions more than I used to.
   2....I have greater difficulty in making decisions than before.
   3...I can't make decisions at all anymore.

2. 0......I can work about as well as I used to.
   1.....It takes an extra effort to get started at doing something.
   2....I have to push myself very hard to do anything.
   3...I can't do any work at all.

3. 0......I can sleep as well as usual.
   1.....I don't sleep as well as I used to.
   2....I wake up 1–2 hours earlier than usual and find it hard to get back to sleep.
   3...I wake up several hours earlier than I used to and cannot get back to sleep.

4. 0......I don't get more tired than usual.
   1.....I get tired more easily than I used to.
   2....I get tired from doing almost nothing.
   3...I am too tired to do anything.

5. 0......My appetite is no worse than usual.
   1.....My appetite is not as good as it used to be.
   2....My appetite is much worse now.
   3...I have no appetite at all anymore.

*Reprinted with permission from LN Matheson. Symptom Magnification Syndrome: Behavioral Medicine Profile. Presented at the Roy Matheson and Associates Work and Assessment Systems Workshop; May 28–31, 1992; Pittsburgh.

6. 0......I haven't lost much weight, if any, lately.
    1.....I have lost more than 5 pounds in the past few months.
    2....I have lost more than 10 pounds in the past few months.
    3...I have lost more than 15 pounds in the past few months.

7. 0......I have not noticed any recent change in my interest in sex.
    1.....I am less interested in sex than I used to be.
    2....I am much less interested in sex now.
    3...I have lost interest in sex completely.

8. 0......My job future is very secure.
    1.....My job future is uncertain but I am hopeful.
    2....My job future is uncertain and I am pessimistic about my prospects.
    3...I don't think I will ever work again.

9. 0......My responsibilities are the same as before my injury and I am handling them well.
    1.....My responsibilities are less than before my injury and I am handling them well.
    2....My responsibilities are less than before my injury and I am struggling.
    3...My responsibilities are overwhelming me.

10. 0......When I am working, I get a lot of satisfaction out of my work.
    1.....When I am working, I get some satisfaction out of my work.
    2....When I am working, I get little satisfaction out of my work.
    3...When I am working, I get no satisfaction out of my work.

11. 0......I am always able to control my symptoms.
    1.....I am able to control my symptoms in most situations.
    2....I am able to control my symptoms in some situations.
    3...My symptoms are not under my control.

12. 0......My symptoms don't restrict me in any way.
    1.....My symptoms restrict me in some activities.
    2....My symptoms restrict me in many activities.
    3...My symptoms restrict me in almost all activities.

13. 0......This injury hasn't had any long-term effect on my life.
    1.....This injury has affected my life in some small but important ways.
    2....This injury has affected my life in many important ways.
    3...This injury has destroyed my life and much of what is important to me.

14. 0......I know what will make my pain worse and can control it.
    1.....I usually know what will make my pain worse but sometimes can't control it.
    2....I sometimes know what will make my pain worse but often can't control my pain.
    3...I don't know what makes my pain worse and it's usually out of control.

15. I am purposely trying to lose weight by eating less: Yes   No

How are you feeling?

Please read each of the following groups of statements carefully. Then pick out the one statement in each group that best describes the way you have been feeling **during the past week, including today!** Circle the number beside the statement you have chosen.

1. 0......I do not feel sad.
   1.....I feel sad.
   2....I am sad all the time and I can't snap out of it.
   3...I am so sad or unhappy that I can't stand it.

2. 0......I am not particularly discouraged about the future.
   1.....I feel discouraged about the future.
   2....I feel I have nothing to look forward to.
   3...I feel the future is hopeless and that things cannot improve.

3. 0......I do not feel like a failure.
   1.....I feel I have failed more than the average person.
   2....As I look back on my life, all I can see is a lot of failure.
   3...I feel I am a complete failure as a person.

4. 0......I get as much satisfaction out of things as I used to.
   1.....I don't enjoy things the way I used to.
   2....I don't get real satisfaction out of anything anymore.
   3...I am dissatisfied or bored with everything.

5. 0......I don't feel particularly guilty.
   1.....I feel guilty a good part of the time.
   2....I feel quite guilty most of the time.
   3...I feel guilty all of the time.

6. 0......I don't feel I am being punished.
   1.....I feel I may be punished.
   2....I expect to be punished.
   3...I feel I am being punished.

7. 0......I don't feel disappointed in myself.
   1.....I am disappointed in myself.
   2....I am disgusted with myself.
   3...I hate myself.

8. 0......I don't feel I am any worse than anyone else.
   1.....I am critical of myself for my weaknesses or faults.
   2....I blame myself all the time for my faults.
   3...I blame myself for everything bad that happens.

9. 0......I don't have thoughts of killing myself.
   1.....I have thoughts of killing myself, but I would not carry them out.
   2....I would like to kill myself.
   3...I would kill myself if I had the chance.

10. 0......I don't cry any more than usual.
    1.....I cry more now than I used to.
    2....I cry all the time now.
    3...I used to be able to cry, but now I don't cry even though I want to.

11. 0......I am no more irritated now than I ever was.
    1.....I get annoyed or irritated more easily than I used to.
    2....I feel irritated all the time now.
    3...I don't get irritated at all by the things that used to irritate me.

12. 0......I have not lost interest in other people.
    1.....I am less interested in other people than I used to be.
    2....I have lost most of my interest in other people.
    3...I have lost all of my interest in other people.

13. 0......I don't look worse than I used to.
    1.....I am worried that I am looking unattractive.
    2....There are changes in my appearance that make me look unattractive.
    3...I believe that I look ugly.

14. 0......I am no more worried about my health than usual.
    1.....I am worried about my physical problems.
    2....I am so worried about my physical problems that it's hard to think of much else.
    3...I am so worried about my physical problems that I cannot think about anything else.

15. 0......I am not angry or upset about my injury.
    1.....I sometimes am angry and upset about my injury.
    2....I frequently am angry and upset about my injury.
    3...I am so angry and upset about my injury that I cannot think about anything else.

You and your job

We are interested in how this injury has affected your ability to work outside the home. Please carefully read and respond to the following questions:

1. Before your injury, were you working outside the home?
      Full-time? _____
      Part-time? _____

2. Are you working outside the home now?
      Yes, full-time in my regular job _____
      Yes, part-time in my regular job _____
      Yes, full-time in a new job _____
      Yes, part-time in a new job _____
      No, I am not working outside the home _____

If you are working, we have no further questions. If you are not now working, please respond to the following two questions.

3. Within the next month
   I expect to return to work   I do not expect to return to work
      |___|___|___|___|___|___|___|___|___|___|

4. Within the next 6 months
   I expect to return to work   I do not expect to return to work
      |___|___|___|___|___|___|___|___|___|___|

Behavioral Medicine Profile Summary and Analysis
Employment and Rehabilitation Institute of California
Leonard N. Matheson, Ph.D.

Name: _____ **Date:** _____

Goals
____A: Keep working or get back to work   Goal rating ____
____B: Get rid of my pain
____C: Resume activities that are important to me
____D: Get my pain under control

Function/Activity Adjustment
1 _____/_____   Interpretation:
2_____/ _____
3_____/ _____
Total _____

Affect/Emotional Adjustment
1_____/ _____   Interpretation:
2_____/ _____
3_____/ _____
Total _____

Suicide risk
1 = Low; 5 = High: _____

Return-to-work expectations
Within the next month
|_____|_____|_____|_____|_____|_____|_____|_____|_____|_____|_____|
Within the next six months
|_____|_____|_____|_____|_____|_____|_____|_____|_____|_____|_____|

Intervention recommended

By: _____**Date:** _____

Behavioral Medicine Profile Instructions for Scoring
Employment and Rehabilitation Institute of California
Leonard N. Matheson, Ph.D.

The Employment and Rehabilitation Institute of California has developed a Behavioral Medicine Profile (BMP) to perform a brief screening of individuals who have been disabled due to a physical injury or illness for 3 months or longer. Items in the BMP are based on the Beck Depression Inventory and the Symptom Results Questionnaire. Some of the items have been modified to address the issues presented by individuals who experience chronic disabling pain.

The BMP was designed to be used within the context of a multidisciplinary work hardening team. In typical use, the patient completes the BMP before an intake interview, which is undertaken by a physician, physical therapist, occupational therapist, vocational specialist, or rehabilitation nurse. The BMP is reviewed during the intake interview and is subsequently scored by a clerk. After scoring, the BMP is provided to the team psychologist for review. The BMP is used within the following guidelines:

1. Every "3" response is investigated by interview with a professional team member. If a satisfactory response is not received, referral to the team psychologist for an informal interview is initiated.

2. Any score of other than "0" on Item 9 under "How are you feeling?" is reviewed with the patient by a psychologist. This may be on an informal basis but should be thoroughly reviewed.

3. A score of 14 or greater on the "How are you doing?" section requires an informal interview with a psychologist.

4. A score of 15 or more on the "How are you feeling?" section requires an informal interview with a psychologist.

Based on these criteria, the BMP will usually trigger appropriate team responses. At the very least, every BMP will be reviewed by the team psychologist and may trigger an informal interview by the psychologist. If responses to the BMP trigger a formal evaluation, the psychologist should confer with his or her team, referring professional, and the patient's insurance carrier before proceeding with a formal evaluation. The formal evaluation by the psychologist will address the issues raised in the BMP.

The sections on "What are your goals?" and "You and your job" are routinely reviewed by clinical staff. The optimal goal rating is shown on the Profile Summary and Analysis. Goal ratings are as follows:

"Positive" goals	"Negative" goals
A = 1	A = 4
B = 4	B = 1
C = 2	C = 3
D = 3	D = 2

These ratings can be used by the team to challenge the patient to develop an appropriate future orientation. At the very least, they should be reviewed as part of the intake interview. It may also be of use to review these items before discharging the patient.

Appendix 3-6
Oswestry Low Back Pain Disability Questionnaire*

Name: _____ **Chart No.:** _____
Occupation: _____ **Date:** _____

How long have you had back pain? _____ Years _____ Months _____ Weeks
How long have you had leg pain? _____ Years ____ Months _____ Weeks

Please read:
This questionnaire has been designed to give us information as to how your back pain has affected your ability to manage in everyday life. Please answer every section, and circle in each section only the **one choice that applies to you.** We realize you may consider that two of the statements in any one section relate to you, but please **circle only the number that most closely describes your problem.**

Section 1: Pain intensity	Section 2: Personal care (washing, dressing, etc.)
0. I can tolerate the pain I have without having to use pain killers. 1. The pain is bad but I manage without taking pain killers. 2. Pain killers give complete relief from pain. 3. Pain killers give moderate relief from pain. 4. Pain killers give very little relief from pain. 5. Pain killers have no effect on the pain and I do not use them.	0. I can look after myself normally without causing extra pain. 1. I can look after myself normally but it causes extra pain. 2. It is painful to look after myself and I am slow and careful. 3. I need some help but manage most of my personal care. 4. I need help every day in most aspects of self care. 5. I do not get dressed, wash with difficulty, and stay in bed.

Section 3: Lifting	Section 4: Walking
0. I can lift heavy weights without extra pain. 1. I can lift heavy weights but it gives extra pain. 2. Pain prevents me from lifting heavy weights off the floor, but I can manage if they are conveniently positioned—for example, on a table. 3. Pain prevents me from lifting heavy weights but I can manage light to medium weights if they are conveniently positioned. 4. I can lift only very light weights. 5. I cannot lift or carry anything at all.	0. Pain does not prevent me from walking any distance. 1. Pain prevents me from walking more than 1 mile. 2. Pain prevents me from walking more than ½ of a mile. 3. Pain prevents me from walking more than ¼ of a mile. 4. I can only walk using a stick or crutches.

*Reprinted with permission from JCT Fairbank, J Couper, JB Davies, UP O'Brien. The Oswestry low back pain disability questionnaire. Physiotherapy 1980;66(8):271.

Section 5: Sitting	Section 6: Standing
0. I can sit in any chair as long as I like. 1. I can only sit in my favorite chair as long as I like. 2. Pain prevents me sitting more than 1 hour. 3. Pain prevents me from sitting more than 30 minutes. 4. Pain prevents me from sitting more than 10 minutes. 5. Pain prevents me from sitting at all.	0. I can stand as long as I want without extra pain. 1. I can stand as long as I want but it gives me extra pain. 2. Pain prevents me from standing for more than 1 hour. 3. Pain prevents me from standing for more than 30 minutes. 4. Pain prevents me from standing for more than 10 minutes. 5. Pain prevents me from standing at all.
Section 7: Sleeping	**Section 8: Sex life**
0. Pain does not prevent me from sleeping well. 1. I can sleep well only by using tablets. 2. Even when I take tablets I have less than 6 hours of sleep. 3. Even when I take tablets I have less than 4 hours of sleep. 4. Even when I take tablets I have less than 2 hours of sleep. 5. Pain prevents me from sleeping at all.	0. My sex life is normal and causes no extra pain. 1. My sex life is normal but causes some extra pain. 2. My sex life is nearly normal but is very painful. 3. My sex life is severely restricted by pain. 4. My sex life is nearly absent because of pain. 5. Pain prevents any sex life at all.
Section 9: Social life	**Section 10: Traveling**
0. My social life is normal and gives me no extra pain. 1. My social life is normal but increases the degree of pain. 2. Pain has no significant effect on my social life apart from limiting my more energetic interests (e.g., dancing, etc). 3. Pain has restricted my social life and I do not go out as often. 4. Pain has restricted my social life to my home. 5. I have no social life because of pain.	0. I can travel anywhere without extra pain. 1. I can travel anywhere but it gives me extra pain. 2. Pain is bad but I mange journeys of more than 2 hours. 3. Pain restricts me to journeys of less than 1 hour. 4. Pain restricts me to short necessary journeys of less than 30 minutes. 5. Pain prevents me from traveling except to the doctor or hospital.

Comments _____

_____

_____

_____

_____

The Oswestry Low Back Pain Disability
Questionnaire Score Interpretation

Each section is scored on a scale of 0–5, with 5 indicating the greatest disability. The scores for all sections are added together (with a maximum score of 50). The final score is expressed as a percentage, with the patients' score being divided by the maximum possible score (based on the number of sections answered).

0–20%: Minimal disability

This group can cope with most living activities. Usually no treatment is indicated, apart from advice on lifting, sitting posture, physical fitness, and diet. Some patients have particular difficulty with sitting, and this may be important if their occupation is sedentary—for example, a typist or driver.

20–40%: Moderate disability

This group experiences more pain and problems with sitting, lifting, and standing. Travel and social life are more difficult, and those in this group may well be off work. Personal care, sexual activity, and sleeping are not grossly affected, and the back condition can usually be managed by conservative means.

40–60%: Severe disability

Pain remains the main problem in this group of patients, but travel, personal care, social life, sexual activity, and sleep are also affected. These patients require detailed investigation.

60–80%: Crippled

Back pain impinges on all aspects of these patients' lives both at home and at work, and positive intervention is required.

80–100%

These patients are either bed-bound or exaggerating their symptoms. This can be evaluated by careful observation of the patient during the medical examination.

Appendix 3-7

The McGill Pain Questionnaire*

Patient's name: _____ **Age:** _____

File number: _____ **Date:** _____

Clinical category (e.g., cardiac, neurologic, etc.): _____

Diagnosis: _____

_____

_____

Analgesic (if already administered):
1. Type: _____
2. Dosage: _____
3. Time given in relation to this test: _____

Patient's intelligence: circle number that represents best estimate

   1 (low)   2   3   4   5 (high)

This questionnaire has been designed to tell us more about your pain.
Four major questions we ask are
1. Where is your pain?
2. What does it feel like?
3. How does it change with time?
4. How strong is it?

It is important that you tell us how your pain feels now. Please follow the instructions at the beginning of each part.

Part 1. Where is your pain? Please mark on the drawings below the areas where you feel pain. Put E if external or I if internal near the areas you mark. Put EI if both external and internal.

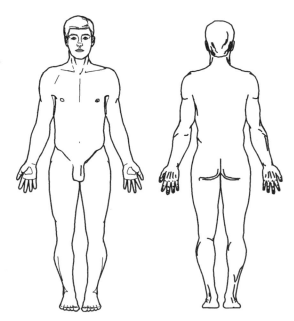

*Reprinted with permission from R Melzack. The McGill Pain Questionnaire: major properties and scoring methods. Pain 1975;1:277.

Part 2. What does your pain feel like?
Some of the words below describe your *present* pain. Mark only those words that best describe it. Leave out any category that is not suitable. Use only a single word in each appropriate category—the one that best applies.

1. Flickering ____ Quivering ____ Pulsing ____ Throbbing ____ Beating ____ Pounding ____	2. Jumping ____ Flashing ____ Shooting ____ Stabbing ____ Lancinating ____	3. Pricking ____ Boring ____ Drilling ____	4. Sharp ____ Cutting ____ Lacerating ____
5. Pinching ____ Pressing ____ Gnawing ____ Cramping ____ Crushing ____	6. Tugging ____ Pulling ____ Wrenching ____ Searing ____	7. Hot ____ Burning ____ Scalding ____ Stinging ____	8. Tingling ____ Itchy ____ Smarting ____
9. Dull ____ Sore ____ Hurting ____ Aching ____ Heavy ____	10. Tender ____ Taut ____ Rasping ____	11. Tiring ____ Exhausting ____ Aching ____	12. Sickening ____ Suffocating ____ Splitting ____
13. Fearful ____ Frightful ____ Terrifying ____	14. Punishing ____ Grueling ____ Cruel ____ Vicious ____ Killing ____	15. Wretched ____ Blinding ____	16. Annoying ____ Troublesome ____ Miserable ____ Intense ____ Unbearable ____
17. Spreading ____ Radiating ____ Penetrating ____ Piercing ____	18. Tight ____ Numb ____ Drawing ____ Squeezing ____ Tearing ____	19. Cool ____ Cold ____ Freezing ____	20. Nagging ____ Nauseating ____ Agonizing ____ Dreadful ____ Torturing ____

Part 3. How does your pain change with time?

1. Which word or words would you use to describe the **pattern** of your pain?

1	2	3
Continuous	Rhythmic	Brief
Steady	Periodic	Momentary
Constant	Intermittent	Transient

2. What kind of things **relieve** your pain?

_____

3. What kind of things **increase** your pain?

_____

Appendix 3-8

Roland and Morris Disability Questionnaire*

When your back hurts, you may find it difficult to do some of the things you normally do. This list contains some sentences that people have used to describe themselves when they have back pain. When you read them, you may find that some stand out because they describe you today. As you read the list, think of yourself today. When you read a sentence that describes you today, put a tick after it. If the sentence does not describe you, then don't mark the sentence and go on to the next one. Remember, tick the sentence only if you are sure that it describes you today.

1. I stay at home most of the time because of my back.
2. I change positions frequently to try and get my back comfortable.
3. I walk more slowly than usual because of my back.
4. Because of my back I am not doing any of the jobs that I usually do around the house.
5. Because of my back, I use a handrail to get upstairs.
6. Because of my back, I lie down to rest more often.
7. Because of my back, I have to hold on to something to get out of an easy chair.
8. Because of my back, I try to get other people to do things for me.
9. I get dressed more slowly than usual because of my back.
10. I only stand up for short periods of time because of my back.
11. Because of my back, I try not to bend or kneel down.
12. I find it difficult to get out of a chair because of my back.
13. My back is painful almost all the time.
14. I find it difficult to turn over in bed because of my back.
15. My appetite is not very good because of my back pain.
16. I have trouble putting on my socks (or stockings) because of the pain in my back.
17. I walk only short distances because of my back pain.
18. I sleep less well because of my back.
19. Because of my back pain, I get dressed with help from someone else.
20. I sit down for most of the day because of my back.
21. I avoid heavy jobs around the house because of my back.
22. Because of my back pain, I am more irritable and bad tempered with people than usual.
23. Because of my back, I go upstairs more slowly than usual.
24. I stay in bed most of the time because of my back.

---

*Reprinted with permission from M Roland, R Morris. A study of the natural history of back pain. Part I: development of a reliable and sensitive measure of disability in low-back pain. Spine 1983;8:141–144.

Patients are given a score of 1 point for each ticked item on the questionnaire. Scores may range from 0 to 24, with a score of zero indicating no disability and a score of 24 indicating severe disability.

4

Postural Dynamics: Functional Causes of Low Back Pain

Richard Jackson

Some schools teach that ideal posture is represented by a plumb line that passes through the ear lobe, the shoulder, just behind the hips, and just in front of the knee and ankle. Two things should be kept in mind. First, plumb lines are rarely available in a clinic. Second, patients never demonstrate ideal posture—that is why they are patients. Even after extensive therapy, a patient still will not demonstrate ideal posture.

So, why learn about postural alignment? How does an individual's posture relate to low back pain (LBP)? These are valid questions, and an attempt will be made in this chapter to give life to the principles of structural alignment.

Everyone can understand the LBP that results from a single injury to the body. It takes the special knowledge of a physical therapist to understand the genesis of the bane of "modern" medicine—chronic recurring LBP. At the root of this understanding is a knowledge of the anatomic, geometric, and kinesiologic factors involved in postural dynamics. It involves how we stand, sit, and move.

Regardless of the activity or inactivity in which an individual is engaged, there are basic rules and principles that must be obeyed for tissue to remain healthy and pain free. When I was taught about posture in school, I heard about plumb lines and the importance of maintaining a lordosis in sitting and that sleeping on your stomach was very, very bad. I learned about ligamentous "creep" and muscle imbalances that occur from poor posture. This material was all very "local," and it proved of limited benefit, clinically. There is more to it. Posture is not static. On the contrary, posture is very dynamic. It is also quite basic.

Physical therapy students graduate from school with all of the pieces they need to put together the mechanical LBP "puzzle." Therapists know and are familiar with each piece of the puzzle. The problem is that they rarely put the pieces together. It is expected that once in the clinic they will put the puzzle together. When they start their first job, they find that there are more patients to be treated than they ever imagined, and they simply do not have time to put the puzzle together. The goal of this chapter is to bring the pieces together.

The basic premise of this material is that the lower half of the body functions as a single unit. It is a linkage system. Each component influences and is influenced by the other components. The human body is a machine; the component motions are predictable, but individual variations do occur. All motion occurs from the integrated function of the individual motion segments of the lower half. Dysfunction of any segment will affect the function of the whole machine. This is a simple concept and is just plain common sense. You will find that the majority of clinicians today ignore this fact and focus only on the area of pain.

Like a machine, the body seeks symmetry and balance. This is consistent with the basic design of the links in the kinetic chain. Herein lies the importance of postural evaluation, both static and dynamic. This evaluation affords you some of your best clues to the root causes of your patient's pain. It is essential that the body be viewed as a whole, and to remember that malalignment or dysfunction of any part will affect the whole.

Unlike a machine made up of nuts and bolts, the human machine has the capacity to compensate when certain areas are malfunctioning. For instance, when a joint is stiff, other joints in the system can compensate or substitute for the lost motion. This can be referred to as the body's adaptive potential. The substitution creates an additional demand both in terms of increasing physical force and increasing metabolic activity. If demand on an area exceeds the tissue's ability to handle that demand, then tissue breakdown will occur. But remember, demand on an area can be increased because dysfunction is present elsewhere.

Force (Stress) Causes Tissue Breakdown

Consider this scenario: Someone is hitting you on the back with a yardstick. Of course, it hurts. Basically, the force acting on the superficial tissues exceeds the tissue's tolerance—that is, a light tap would not hurt. Stopping the pain is simply a matter of stopping the yardstick from hitting the tissue. How do clinicians handle this scenario? By and large, they begin treating the tissue. Herein lies the basic problem in evaluation and treatment of LBP. We are all looking in the wrong direction.

It is force, or stress, that causes tissue to break down. The body's response to tissue breakdown is inflammation. Inflammation excites nociceptors, which bombard the central nervous system (CNS) with afferent impulses. The CNS reads this as pain. Pain comes from tissue breakdown, and persistent pain comes from persistent breakdown. Numerous studies have shown that it is inflammation that causes LBP.[1-3]

It does not matter what structure is involved in generating pain. Therapists need to identify *the forces that caused the tissue to break down.* It does not matter if the pain is coming from the disc, the joints, or the soft tissues. What matters is finding the source of the forces that caused the breakdown and then designing a treatment plan to remove those forces.

The role of the therapist must be to analyze the cause of the pain—that is, to do a complete evaluation to find the source or sources of the destructive forces that are damaging the tissue, and then to outline a treatment plan that will remove this force or these forces without creating further problems. Of course, damaged tissue and the secondary effects of pain, such as muscle tension, may have to be treated locally. This can be looked at as "secondary" treatment. The primary treatment is removal of destructive forces.

One important point when we are discussing tissue breakdown is the definition of normal force—either too much or *too little* force arriving at a tissue can be destructive. Furthermore, there are many factors that can impair a tissue's ability to attenuate force, such as age, previous injury, lifestyle issues (such as smoking), and occupation.

The Low Back Dilemma

In 1990, there were nearly 15 million physician office visits for mechanical LBP. This ranks fifth as a reason for all physician visits, and nearly 25% of these patients were referred for orthopedic consultation.[4]

Back pain is the single most common ailment seen by physical therapists entering orthopedic practice, ranging from 25% to 50% of patient visits. Therapists view disc problems as the primary cause of LBP and the McKenzie method is the most common treatment approach.[5]

Many studies have sought to determine the primary pain generators in the low back. It is now known that the disc is responsible for approximately 36% of back pain cases; facet joints account for 15%, and the sacroiliac joints account for 30%. It is assumed that in the remaining 19% soft tissue, combined lesions, or bones are responsible.[6-8] Everyone is concerned about the "pain generator" and not looking at the forces—or lack thereof—that caused the structure to become a pain generator.

It is generally recognized that the majority of individuals who develop LBP do not need medical intervention. That is probably because of a basic fact about human tissue: It has a tendency to heal when traumatized. So why does some pain remain? Why do some tissues fail to heal?

The following are three possible causes for chronic pain:

1. The trauma, single or cumulative, is so great and the damage so extensive that the tissue cannot repair itself. Torn ligaments, large cartilaginous lesions, and intervertebral disc degeneration are examples of this, as are instabilities.
2. Conditions where chronic pain has been disassociated from the original physical basis. There may be little evidence remaining of a nociceptive stimulus. Waddell[9] described this as chronic illness behavior. This is where chronic pain progressively becomes a self-sustaining condition that is resistant to traditional medical management.
3. A stimulus remains that continues to be destructive to the tissues involved or is preventing the healing process. This is the emphasis of this material.

As physical therapists, we must be able to recognize the cause of chronic pain. Can we help the patient? There are certain conditions that are not amenable to physical therapy. Also, we must be able to discern the signs and symptoms of physical disease from those of distress and illness behavior.[9] Fortunately, the majority of our patients with chronic, recurring LBP are treatable. The main question is, "Where to begin?" Therein lies the identity crisis of the physical therapist. Twenty years ago physical therapists were told that their modalities had the power to heal, and effectiveness was measured by a therapist's skill at selecting the appropriate modality. These days therapists are confused by those who say "mobilize," those who say "stabilize," and those who "theorize" over a "missing link."

Research shows that tissues become healthy with activity and people get better with movement. Physical therapists are movement specialists. The body is a machine, and physical therapists, more than any other professionals, know how the machine works. We are mechanics: Fix the machine as best you can, and then you are done. No magic, no missing links, just nuts and bolts. We are going to stick to some basic principles that we learned in physical therapy school as a basis for treating the most resistant musculoskeletal problem today: chronic LBP.

The Basics

The body is a machine and it follows certain rules. If we obey the rules we stay healthy, if we break the rules then injury will result. Poor posture, either static or dynamic, breaks all the rules. That is why assessment of alignment is so important.

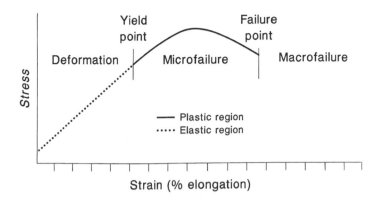

Figure 4-1 Stress-strain curve. Stress on a tissue results in a strain. The maximum tensile deformation of collagen before failure is 6–8%. (Courtesy of R Jackson, PT, OCS.)

Tissue Injury and Repair

Force, either too much or too little, is the cause of injury. The primary forces acting on the body are (1) tension, (2) compression, and (3) shear. When these forces become excessive, tissue damage occurs.

All biological tissue is subjected to a variety of deforming forces every day. These forces may be external or internal and can be defined in terms of force per unit area (stress). This stress produces a resultant strain, or deformation of tissue. Stress and strain can be plotted against one another to gain an understanding of the strength of a particular structure[10–12] (Figure 4-1).

The maximum tensile deformation of collagen before failure is 6–8%. In the first phase of deformation, collagen fibers line up (called the "toe of the curve"). Disruption of connective tissue occurs if the ultimate tensile strength is exceeded. Again, this may be from a single load or a summation of loads.[10–12]

It is important to recognize that a certain amount of stress to tissue is required for tissue to remain healthy. All musculoskeletal tissues derive their health, nutrition, and strength from regular, nondestructive stress, whereas rest and inactivity decrease tissue health.[9,10,13–20] Therefore, tissues need to be stressed but not overstressed. This is graphically demonstrated in Figure 4-2.

A second and very common type of soft-tissue injury results from submaximal stress.[12] Brand has demonstrated that a single strike of 1.5 kg to a finger pad is inconsequential. Several repetitions caused discomfort, and 1,000 or more impacts caused signs of inflammation and pain. This is a clear

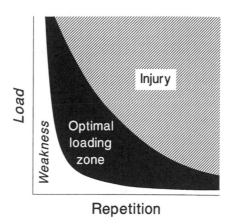

Figure 4-2 Optimal and destructive loading of tissue. All tissue needs an optimal amount of stress to stay healthy. Stress can increase with load or repetitions. Too much or too little force arriving at a tissue can be destructive. (Courtesy of R Jackson, PT, OCS.)

example of cumulative trauma. In another experiment, with repetitions decreased over a prolonged period of time, the tissues were able to accommodate to the stress.[21] Kosiak demonstrated that as the impact force increased, the number of repetitions needed for tissue change to occur decreased.[21] What these studies tell us is quite simple. Tissues are designed to handle a finite amount of stress over time. If the amount of times a force hits the tissue (frequency) is increased or the magnitude of force (load) is increased, then tissue breaks down.

As far as repair of damaged tissue is concerned, the same rules apply—movement is necessary. In fact, numerous studies have shown that exercise is necessary in the rehabilitation of LBP patients.[9,13,16,22–29] The therapist must remember that too much stress in rehabilitation will break down tissue, too little will inhibit restoration of normal tissue function.

Figure 4-2 also illustrates the real meaning of the "plumb line" in postural analysis. Normal function, either static or dynamic, cannot be rigidly prescribed. Essentially, there is a wide range of acceptable "normal" alignment. The goal with a patient is not to achieve the "ideal." The goal is simply to bring the integrated structural unit (i.e., the patient's body) into the optimal loading zone. All things considered, this zone is quite large. The key is to work with the individual dynamics of the patient and devise ways to "tune" the entire system to function within the optimal loading zones.

Joints

Articular cartilage is a highly specialized connective tissue with high tensile strength. It is resistant to shearing and compressive forces and possesses resilience and elasticity.[10]

Articular cartilage forms a thin covering on the joint surfaces. It has two main functions: (1) to aid in dissipating loads applied to the joint, and (2) to minimize friction with motion.

Cartilage consists of approximately 60% water and 40% solid matrix. The solid matrix is 60% collagen and 40% proteoglycan gel. Because of its highly viscoelastic properties, articular cartilage is suited for compressive loading. An increase in physical activity increases the thickness and elasticity of articular cartilage.[11]

There are some fallacies regarding cartilage. Among these are that cartilage is metabolically inactive and unable to repair itself and that cartilage wears out with use. In fact, articular cartilage is a metabolically active tissue, and the synthesis of matrix in an arthritic joint is actually greater than in a noninvolved joint. Reparative cartilage in an involved joint may come from synovium or subchondral bone (extrinsic repair) or may come from the damaged cartilage itself (intrinsic repair). In postmortem studies of damaged joints, evidence of both intrinsic and extrinsic repair can be found. The ability of cartilage to repair itself was recognized by many, but until recently these views were overlooked in the general belief that cartilage was metabolically inactive.[14]

It is important to understand that there is no such thing as a local injury to a joint. When a joint begins to break down, all of the structures of the joint are involved, including synovium, capsule, and ligaments.[14] Furthermore, the chronicity of joint degeneration is not necessarily a failure on the part of joint tissue to repair; rather, the forces that caused the onset of joint degeneration are still present.[14]

Joints are designed to function in mid-range but need regular movement through full range to stay healthy. Because it is avascular, cartilage receives its nutrition from compressive forces. Joints thrive on compressive forces but react adversely to repetitive impulse loading.[30,31] This explains the degenerative effects of frequent loading of a joint that cannot effectively transmit shock because of joint dysfunction. Articulations are not designed to function at end range for prolonged periods of time. In this position, articular cartilage is under prolonged compression and will break down.[31] Most authors ascribe local failure of cartilage to excessive "wear and tear." This is simply not the case *as long as the joint is structurally and biomechanically sound.*

There is evidence that degenerative changes occur in areas of cartilage that are not subject to the alternating pressures of weight bearing. In normal joints, those areas of cartilage that do not articulate with opposed cartilage inevitably become softened (chondromalacia). *The single most important mechanical factor for a healthy joint surface is the quality of movement.*[15,31] Optimal or high quality movement is achieved when joints are stable and have full and unimpeded range of motion with proper load distribution throughout the range.

Postural asymmetries can alter the load distribution on all of the joints in the system. Abnormal loading of joints has been shown to lead to articular degeneration.[32–36] Joint health is dependent on the symmetry and integrity of the individual joint and of all the other joints within the kinetic chain.

All of the cartilaginous structures of the body respond adversely to disuse and prolonged loading and respond positively to movement and exercise. Research has shown that endurance training, such as long duration walking or running, is not associated with premature joint degeneration. In fact, it is strongly associated with overall strengthening of articular structures.[19] Cartilage thrives within a wide range of forces. Constant compression leads to thinning, but it may regain its thickness if the compression is slowly released. It becomes thicker with intermittent compression. Again, excessive compression, such as end-range functioning for a prolonged time, causes degeneration of cartilage.[31]

Normal joint function depends on a number of factors including (1) joint stability, (2) freedom of movement (full range), and (3) proper load distribution through the joint. There is ample evidence that any factor that disturbs the normal symmetry or arthrokinematics in the lower extremities and spine will produce abnormal loading, joint instability, abnormal movement, and therefore articular degeneration.[14,31,37–46]

Even small displacements of bone can markedly alter joint mechanics. For instance, Ramsey and Hamilton[37] have shown that a 1-mm displacement in talar position reduced the contact area of the talus and tibia by 42%. It can easily be seen what effect this will have on the articulation. The impulsive load will increase and quite possibly exceed the optimal load level of the joint. The forces normally acting on articular cartilage must fall within a range suited to the continued vitality and viability of the cells. The forces in the joint must be sufficient to provide nutrition and to stimulate chondrocytes for adequate matrix production. Chondrolysis, or degeneration, will occur when stress on the cartilage falls outside of the optimal loading levels.[14]

Radin and colleagues[30,34,35] demonstrated that one of the factors leading to cartilage degeneration is "repetitive impulsive loading." This is an important concept in understanding joint breakdown, and it is worth taking a moment to understand the underlying etiology.

First, in handling high-magnitude longitudinal forces (as in the spine and lower extremities), the cartilage and synovial fluid have a minimal role in shock absorption. It is the soft tissue and bone that attenuate these forces. Since the nineteenth century, Wolff's law has been used to help us understand the adaptation of tissue, especially osseous tissue, to stress. The internal structure of a bone will change according to the imposed demands. Radin et al.[30,34,35] proposed that when a bone is subjected to repetitive impulse loading, the bone underlying the joint, especially the subchondral bone, remodels and strengthens itself. This will occur when there is joint dysfunction, rendering the joint less effective in transmitting force proximally. The effect of subchondral hardening is to render the subchondral bone less effective in force attenuation, thereby increasing the forces on the cartilage itself. Consider, by way of example, the effect of dropping a load onto your foot. The damage sustained by your foot is related to the amount of weight dropped and to the hardness of the surface underneath your foot. Therefore, normal loading of a joint strengthens it, whereas abnormal loading breaks it down. Abnormal loading can occur when there is joint dysfunction, joint asymmetry, joint instability, and so forth.

Up to this point we have been discussing the effects of forces on cartilage. What about the effects of immobilization? There is conclusive evidence that atrophy and degeneration of articular cartilage and subchondral bone occur with immobilization.[11,47]

It should be clear at this point that the health of our joints is directly dependent on normal arthrokinematics, which dictate load distribution and load transfer. In addition, full range of motion is essential for normal nutrition. Any factor that disrupts this balance of form and function can lead to tissue damage, inflammation, and pain.

Why do joints become symptomatic? To answer this, you must concentrate on form and function. Look at the whole picture and the interrelationships of the links in the kinetic chain. Whatever you do, do not look at a symptomatic joint and evaluate it without concern for the form and function of the other joints in the system.

Intervertebral Disc

The disc is a joint and, as such, the same rules apply in keeping it healthy. It is made to function in mid-range, motion is essential for its health, and it breaks down when it must function for sustained periods at end range. Because symptoms arise from the disc in up to 36% of LBP patients,[6] it is important to understand its structure and function.

An intervertebral disc is essentially avascular.[48,49] Only the outer wall has a blood supply and nerve supply.[49] Therefore, it must receive its nutrition simply by diffusion.[48–51] Also, the exchange of nutrients is slowed because of constant pressure loads and semipermeable interfascial layers. These unfavorable conditions affect primarily the cells of the intervertebral disc. These cells have a half-life of only a few weeks and need to be replaced constantly. A constant exchange of substances—nutrition into the disc and waste products out of the disc—is necessary to ensure an equilibrium between the synthesis of extracellular structural elements and the breaking down of structural elements.[48] A regular loading-unloading cycle promotes the exchange of nutrients into the disc and immobility results in a slow-down of nutrient exchange, even resulting in dehydration.[19,48–51]

One thing that helps us to understand the dynamics of the intervertebral disc is the process of aging and its effect on the disc. There is no question that discs change with age. There is evidence that the degeneration that occurs with aging is related to decreasing nutrition of the central disc. The decreased nutrition allows for an accumulation of waste products (the result of intradiscal cellular breakdown), which results in a fall in pH levels that further accelerates intradiscal breakdown.[52] It is a vicious cycle. The issue is nutrition, and we know that discal nutrition is dependent on full and free spinal motion.

It should be obvious, given the foregoing research regarding the disc, that symmetry and repetitive full-range motion is essential for the health of the disc. Exercises designed to improve nutrition to the disc will help to optimize disc health and have an inverse effect on the detrimental effect of aging on the intervertebral disc.

Farfan[49] and McNally et al.[53] noted that torsional stresses play a major role in degeneration of the disc. The combined forces of compression and rotation tend to cause annular damage. Sustained static loading of the front or back of the disc will also result in dehydration and degeneration.[19,50,51] Also, full-range movements resulting in regular loading and unloading of the disc promote good nutrition.[19,50,51] Again, the disc functions like the other peripheral joint articulations—they are designed to function in mid-range, not end range, and nutrition is based on full ranges of motion. Postures combining compression and rotation must be avoided.

Vertebral Segment

It is difficult to discuss the health of the intervertebral disc without mentioning its relationship to the facet joints. In normal standing, 16% of the force on the vertebral segment is carried by the facet joints. In sitting, the joints do not carry any load.[54] The facet joints stabilize the intervertebral disc against torsion. Farfan[49] suggested that any impairment of the function of the joints may result in a higher risk of disc degeneration. Furthermore, Gotfried[55] demonstrated that a loss of disc height, such as with degeneration, will result in degeneration of the facet joints.

Tripodism of the segment—that is, weight bearing on the disc in the front and on the facet joints in the back—is essential for spinal segmental stability and health. Anything that disrupts this stability, such as quadrant length asymmetry, poor posture, or limited spinal motion, may have disastrous consequences on the health of the segmental components.

Quadrant Length

Leg Length Discrepancy and Low Back Pain

Symmetry of the right and left lower quadrants is essential in maintaining a healthy and pain-free lower half. This concept, more than any other, is the most difficult to get across to the medical community. There is a fallacy in medicine that leg length discrepancies of less than 1 inch are not significant. This is not supported by research. Before reviewing the literature, however, see Figure 4-3.

Considering the basic rules of joint health outlined earlier in the chapter, it is obvious that leg length inequality causes articulations of the spine and lower extremities to break the rules required for healthy joints.

First, the articulations are no longer symmetric; therefore, they are not functioning in the range for which they were designed. This creates abnormally high impact loading throughout the joints of the system. Furthermore, the spinal segments have lost tripodism and are therefore unstable. The discs are under the combined forces of compression and rotation, which is another unhealthy situation. The facets are sustaining an end-range posture and are unable to undergo a full range of motion. All things considered, quadrant length asymmetry appears to be a potential disaster. Is it? The answer is found in numerous controlled studies.

Giles and Taylor[40] looked at individuals with chronic LBP who also had leg length discrepancies greater than 9 mm. In general, 7% of the adult population with no history of LBP has a leg length inequality greater than 9 mm. Giles found that in groups of patients with chronic LBP, the incidence of discrepancies of 9 mm or more ranged from 13% to 22%.

Subotnick,[43] in a sample of 4,000 symptomatic athletes, found nearly 40% had limb length discrepancies, and there appeared to be a high correlation of injury on the short side and associated weakness. Perennou[56] found that scoliosis was revealed on x-ray films by reports of LBP in 86% of adult cases. Lumbar scoliosis is often associated with leg length dis-

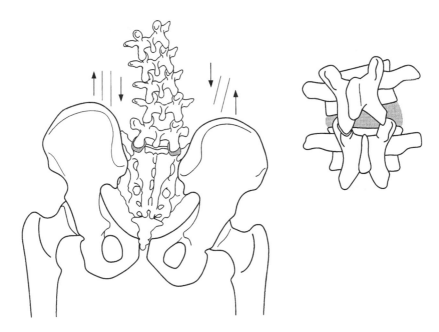

Figure 4-3 Structural compensation in a long left leg. The arrows and parallel lines represent the resulting asymmetries and forces acting at the sacroiliac joints. Leg length discrepancies abnormally load all joints in the system. (Courtesy of R Jackson, PT, OCS.)

crepancies (LLDs). Sicuranza et al.[39] reported on a series of patients who manifested what they called a short-leg syndrome. These are cases of back pain radiating to either leg caused by LLDs and relieved by the use of a heel lift. In addition, Schuit et al.[42] reported success in using a heel lift to restore normal pelvic alignment in the successful treatment of LBP caused by LLDs.

Probably the most compelling work that illustrates the role of LLDs in the development of chronic LBP has been done by Friberg.[57] He pointed out that an LLD is compensated for in the lumbar spine by a functional scoliosis, the concavity being on the long leg side. He cited electromyographic (EMG) investigations by Taillard and Morscher that showed an asymmetric increase in activity of several muscle groups making it impossible for an individual to maintain a resting standing position. Friberg reported that the disc on the concave side is under compression and bulges laterally. A segment in side bending also rotates axially, thereby creating the conditions that promote disc degeneration.[49,53] Tables 4-1 and 4-2 show the results of Friberg's investigation.

Table 4-1 The Incidence of Leg Length Discrepancies in 653 Patients with Chronic Low Back Pain and in 359 Symptom-Free Conscript Soldiers

Leg length inequality (mm)	Low back pain patients' group		Symptom-free control group	
	Number	*Percent*	*Number*	*Percent*
0–4	161	24.6	203	56.5
5–9	296	45.3	100	27.9
10–14	120	18.4	48	13.4
15 or more	76	11.7	8	2.2
Total	653	100.0	359	100.0

Source: Reprinted with permission from O Friberg. Clinical symptoms and biomechanics of lumbar spine and hip joint in leg length inequality. Spine 1983;8:646.

Table 4-2 The Relative Incidence of Leg Length Discrepancies in a Group of Chronic Low Back Pain Patients and in a Group of Symptom-Free Conscripts

Leg Length Inequality (mm)	Low back pain patients' group (p%)	Symptom free control group (c%)	Ratio [(p%) : (c%)]
Less than 5 mm	24.6	56.5	0.43
5 mm or more	75.4	43.5	1.73
10 mm or more	30.1	15.6	1.93
15 mm or more	11.7	2.2	5.32

Source: Reprinted with permission from O Friberg. Clinical symptoms and biomechanics of lumbar spine and hip joint in leg length inequality. Spine 1983;8:646.

Tables 4-1 and 4-2 show that an LLD of 5 mm or more was found in 75.4% of the patients and 43.5% of the controls. The difference was highly significant ($P < .0001$). An LLD of 5 mm or more was 1.73 times greater in the symptomatic group and an LLD of 15 mm or more was 5.32 times that of the symptom-free group.

Friberg reported excellent results when using a shoe lift to treat low back symptoms arising from LLDs. Furthermore, in the group of patients with an LLD of 5 mm or more ($n = 228$), sciatic pain radiated into the longer leg 78.5% of the time and into the shorter leg 21.5% of the time. Also, hip pain and arthrosis occurred on the long side in 89% (226 of 254 patients) and on the short leg side in 11% ($n = 28$). These results of hip arthrosis on the long side agree with the work of Gofton,[45] who further stated that three out of four patients who experience hip bursitis have a long leg on the side of the bursitis. In another investigation, Gofton and Trueman[58] studied 67 patients with osteoarthritis of the hip and found 41 (61%) of these were unilateral. Furthermore, 36 of the 41 had LLDs, and 29 of these patients had osteoarthrosis on the long leg side.

Structural Changes with Leg Length Discrepancy

Numerous structural changes are associated with LLDs. In comparing 100 radiographs of patients with chronic LBP, which included 50 with LLDs greater than 9 mm and 50 with straight spines, Giles and Taylor[44] noted wedging of the fifth lumbar vertebra on anteroposterior views and lateral "traction" spurs and osteophytes, which were common, more frequent, and larger on scoliotic vertebral margins.

It is suggested by the early appearance of traction spurs that asymmetric degeneration occurs at the intervertebral discs when they are stretched at the convexity and compressed on the concavity of the scoliosis. The degenerative changes seen on radiographs showing postural scoliosis caused by LLDs suggest motion segment instability.[44] As stated previously, loss of essential tripodism of the vertebral segment causes instability.

In scoliosis, the forces of deformation first affect the ligaments and muscles. These structures will shorten on the concavity and lengthen on the convexity.[31] Left in this position, these viscoelastic structures will adapt to the new length. Muscles on the concave side will actually shorten, losing sarcomeres and adapting their function to this new position. The muscles on the convex side will also adapt in a similar manner. These changes will need to be addressed in the therapeutic plan when treating individuals who have back pain as a result of a LLD.

Another change consistent with scoliosis is that cartilage degenerates secondary to heavy compression on the concave side. Because there is a lack of compression on the convex side, poor nutrition and degeneration occur. The disc, as previously mentioned, is compressed on the concavity and bulges toward the convexity, thereby rendering the disc incapable of functioning with normal mechanics and fostering conditions conducive to degeneration.[19,31,49,53]

Muscles

The three basic principles of muscle function are (1) resting tension, (2) length tension relationships, and (3) biomechanics of muscle.

Resting Tension

Resting tension of a muscle can be centrally or peripherally controlled. The muscle spindle has a primary role in determining resting tension. The efferent messages sent to the muscle by the CNS determine resting tension. The efferent output to the muscles is directly related to the afferent input from the receptor system (muscle spindle). If the afferent input increases, the efferent output increases. Two common factors that increase muscle tension are environmental stress and pain.

Environmental stress can be a physical or emotional response to a job, family, or surroundings, causing an excitatory response to muscles, which thereby increase the resting muscle tension. Therapists find that people who have generalized "muscle tension" are more difficult to treat and recover more slowly.

Pain is a common cause of increased resting muscle tension. When nociceptors are stimulated, they bombard the CNS with afferent impulses, which are read by the brain as "pain." The reflex efferent response is to increase the "set point" of resting muscle tension. This creates increased resistance passively to any functionally induced length change (Figure 4-4).

One purpose of increased tension is to inhibit motion. This is helpful initially because rest is often indicated for a short time after injury for tissue healing to begin. Problems arise when movement is suppressed for too long, because hard and soft tissues need movement for health and viability. Also, when pain subsides, it does not necessarily follow that the muscles involved will automatically return to their original resting tension. Furthermore, it must be understood that when a muscle is stretched past its resting length, there is a passive resistance to the length change[10,59] (see Figure 4-4). These basic concepts about resting tension lead us into a brief review of the muscle spindle and the gamma efferent system.

The musculoskeletal system is the most massive body system. It receives the most efferent outflow from the CNS. The majority of this outflow is to the muscles. Also, the musculoskeletal system is the main source of input to the CNS. This means that the musculoskeletal system has a dominant influence on the whole person. It therefore follows that disturbances in sensory input from the musculoskeletal system will greatly disturb the individual as an integrated unit.[60]

The feedback mechanism from the peripheral receptors supplies the central system with billions of messages that report on the "state of the system," and the central system responds to the periphery, our joints and muscles, with billions of commands, adjustments, and actions that allow the musculoskeletal system to function. All of this occurs unconsciously. The simple acts of standing up from a chair, picking up a newspaper, and

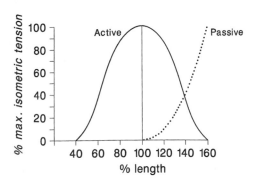

Figure 4-4 Length-tension relationship. Tension in a muscle can be caused by active contraction or passive lengthening. (Courtesy of R Jackson, PT, OCS.)

walking up the stairs require an inconceivable, almost infinite number of sensory and motor impulses to get the job done. It boggles the mind to even consider what has unconsciously and reflexly occurred in these simple acts, let alone in complex acts.

It is healthy for physical therapists to consider such matters because it cannot help but be a humbling experience. It helps to bring into perspective the limits of our knowledge. If we cannot grasp the neuromotor entirety of the act of standing up from a seated position, we cannot begin to understand the effects our treatment procedures have on our patients' daily lives.

Sensory, or afferent, messages are sent to the CNS from an array of receptors in joints, muscles, and other tissues to alert the CNS regarding the condition of the peripheral system. The CNS processes these data and uses them, mostly reflexively, to make adjustments in the peripheral system, via the anterior horn, to keep the body in balance, harmony, and "good working order."

It must be clearly understood that the primary determinant of joint function is muscle function. Farfan[61] pointed out that joints are essentially inert compared with their muscular brethren. A joint is functionally dependent on the muscular system. The function of each muscle is dependent on a variety of factors, including resting length and length-tension relationships. Shortening the resting length of a muscle will result in associated joint motion dysfunction. Joint function is dependent on muscle function[60,61]; therefore, if muscle function is impaired, the joint function will also be impaired.

The majority of *spinal articular* or *peripheral articular* restrictions are muscular in nature. This is the basis of the spinal lesion. It is primarily mus-

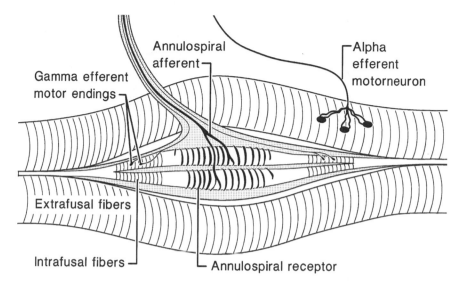

Gamma efferent
motor endings

Annulospiral
afferent

Alpha
efferent
motorneuron

Extrafusal fibers

Intrafusal fibers

Annulospiral receptor

Figure 4-5 The muscle spindle. Contraction of the intrafusal fibers by the gamma efferents will distort the annulospiral endings, causing an extrafusal contraction. Extrafusal lengthening passively will also stimulate the annulospiral receptors, causing a reflex increase in tension of the extrafusal muscle fibers. (Courtesy of R Jackson, PT, OCS.)

cular in nature and that muscular problem is a restriction in *resistance-free lengthening* of muscles. One primary goal in physical therapy is the normalization of resting muscle tension and length. Normalization of these factors is critical for normal joint function. Joint dysfunction is primarily muscular dysfunction, not just a dysfunction of the articular elements. Resting muscle tension is largely dependent on the activity of the muscle spindle. The increase or decrease in resting tension of a muscle is directly related to the increase or decrease in muscle spindle activity.

The neuroanatomy of the muscle spindle is simplified in Figure 4-5. Each spindle is built around three to ten intrafusal muscle fibers that are attached at their ends to the sheaths of the surrounding extrafusal (skeletal muscle) fibers. The intrafusal fibers are interrupted in their middle by a heavily nucleated, noncontractile tissue. Entwined around this central region are the sensory nerve endings of the spindle called the annulospiral receptors. These receptors feed information back to the CNS about the internal state of the muscle spindle.

The intrafusal fibers are innervated by gamma motor neurons, which constitute fully one-third of all ventral horn outflow.[60] The extrafusal fibers are innervated by alpha motor neurons. The muscle spindles exist through-out all skeletal muscle tissue to detect the degree of muscle contraction. They are responsible for the inherent resting tone of all skeletal muscle tissue. The muscle spindle can be stimulated in two ways. First, an increase in gamma efferent outflow from the ventral horn will cause the intrafusal muscle fibers to contract, thereby stretching the annulospiral endings. This results in an afferent bombardment to the cord and a reflex alpha efferent discharge to the muscle, causing it to contract. The purpose of this mechanism is to keep the length relationship of the intrafusal fibers to the extrafusal fibers constant.

A second way to stimulate the muscle spindle is to stretch or lengthen the entire muscle. This causes a stretch of the spindle, stimulating the annulospiral afferents, and the exact same response ensues. The muscle spindle with its gamma efferent motor fibers is essentially a servo control system.[62] This allows the spindle to indirectly control muscle contraction. The spindle, via its sensory receptors, can directly control muscle contraction without impulses having to come from the brain to the anterior horn cell. The gamma system allows muscles to contract reflexively to a predetermined length. This mechanism allows for unconscious control of postural muscles. Too much extension lengthens the flexors and results in a flexor response to maintain alignment, and vice versa.

It is the gamma system that is the primary controller of spindle sensitivity and activity. An increase in gamma activity will increase the resting tension of a muscle. Many conditions could cause an increase in gamma activity. Among these are stress, response to pain, facilitation of spinal segmental activity such as would occur with a hypermobile segment, or quick length changes of a muscle such as in whiplash. The problem is that when the gamma system is turned up, muscles will further resist passive lengthening.

How does this relate to a patient? One major factor in determining the normal operation of the human machine is the assessment of muscle length. Therapists need to assess which muscles are tight. Muscles that are tight will resist length change during normal range of motion or during gait (see Figure 4-4). Remember, muscles can generate a tension actively or passively. The passive line represents resistance to length change. Essentially, tight muscles compromise movement, which will compromise joint nutrition and health.

The important point that is often overlooked in muscle length testing is that muscles can be structurally short (morphologically short) or muscles can be short because they are tense (physiologically short). Morphologic restrictions may come from a loss of sarcomeres, scar tissue, or decreased mobility of connective tissue. A muscle that is physiologically short has an increase in gamma efferent output. For whatever reason, the "gamma gain" has been turned up.

The importance of recognizing this difference is absolutely critical when it comes to designing a treatment plan. Failure to distinguish between morphologically short muscles and physiologically short muscles often results in ineffective treatment.

Why is making this distinction so important? Think back to the muscle spindle. A change in the positional relationship of the extrafusal and the intrafusal fibers will cause an increase in muscle tension. Therefore, stretching a physiologically shortened muscle will increase its tension and make the situation worse.

A morphologically short muscle needs to be stretched. This, by the way, is a misnomer, because we are really stretching fascia when we "stretch a muscle." We are not trying to pull sarcomeres apart when we stretch a muscle. The goal of stretching is to lengthen fascia, thereby achieving a gradual increase in the resting length and resistance-free passive lengthening of the muscle.

A physiologically shortened muscle, one in which the "gamma gain" is increased, will resist length change and therefore will test as a short muscle. The appropriate treatment in this case is to inhibit the muscle (usually through a hold-relax or contract-relax maneuver) and then lengthen it *slowly*. These muscles need to be "coaxed" into relaxation and lengthening. They need to be re-educated to achieve a normal set point of resting tension. Stretching these muscles will spell disaster.

Can a muscle be both physiologically *and* morphologically short? Absolutely. In fact, this is very common. The treatment should be obvious. The muscle must first be inhibited and lengthened with internal tension returned to normal. Then, appropriate stretching can be applied.

Physical therapists can determine the difference between morphologic and physiologic shortening by palpation. Therapists who have had any contact with patients have developed a feel for muscle tension. A second method is to always precede muscle stretching with a *gentle* contract-relax maneuver followed by lengthening. The therapist should continue this technique until there is no longer a gain in length, then a stretch should *gradually* be applied.

This entire discussion leads us back to basic science. Basic science must be applied in clinical practice to achieve the desired result.

Length-Tension Relationships

Muscle includes contractile and elastic components. The contractile component is, of course, the sarcomere, with its actin and myosin filaments. The elastic component is the investing fascia and also the inher-

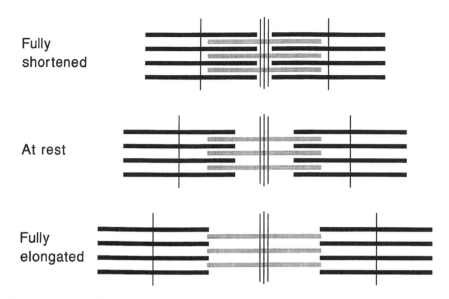

Fully
shortened

At rest

Fully
elongated

Figure 4-6 Length-tension relationship at the sarcomere level. The optimal length to generate maximum tension is resting length. A fully shortened or elongated sarcomere is not able to generate tension. (Courtesy of R Jackson, PT, OCS.)

ent resting tension of the muscle.[59] These elastic components create an elastic resistance to change of length when a muscle is elongated beyond its resting length. The classic length-tension diagram is a graphic depiction of the influence of these components on muscle function (see Figure 4-4).

A muscle can generally produce the maximum amount of contraction at its resting length. If the length of a muscle varies by 60% above or below resting length, active contraction drops to zero[59] (see Figures 4-4 and 4-6).

These basic principles are important when applied to daily function. The muscles used to walk will have an *optimal length* at the moment in gait where they have to generate *optimal strength* and *efficiency*. Changes in the symmetry of the body from its original design, such as postural defects or quadrant length asymmetry, will influence the muscle's ability to act efficiently. Such postural or quadrant length asymmetries eventually result in muscle length and strength deficits. Also, an increase in the resting tension of a muscle will create increased resistance of that muscle to lengthening. This can have a significant influence on gait.

We know that substitutions will occur during gait when there are length (range) or strength deficits.[63–66] Also, muscles that have an increased resting tension, or are adaptively shortened, have a new resting length. Therefore, a muscle's ability to produce a maximum contractile force now occurs at a different point in the range of motion than originally intended. A muscle that has shortened is also a muscle that is functionally weak.

Let us look at an individual with an LLD and consider the muscle problems created concerning length-tension relationships. We know that a long left leg creates a spine in left sidebend, right rotation. The left hip is adducted, the right abducted. We know that the ilium on the left will be posteriorly rotated and the right ilium anteriorly rotated.[41] What types of muscle problems will be created (Figure 4-7)?

The muscles in the frontal plane show a predictable pattern of change. The left erector spinae and multifidus will be short; they have actually lost sarcomeres and are truly short when compared with the right side. The left abductors are long, the right short. The right adductors are long and the left are short. What the illustration does not show is the sagittal and transverse plane muscles. Predictable changes in actual muscle length will occur there as well.

Given the preceding discussion, what will occur when the patient is given a shoe lift to make the quadrants symmetric? Based on what we know about length-tension relationships, all muscles in the triplane system will become functionally weak. In an attempt to help restore symmetry to the body, we actually worsen the condition functionally.

So, what is the answer? The answer is *to think*. While attempting to "fix the machine," always keep in mind the consequences on the machine of the intervention. In the example given, triplanar functional exercises obviously must be given to the patient in order to *complete* the treatment. Also, give the patient time to adapt.

Biomechanics of Muscle

Muscles move joints by a contractile force acting at a distance from that joint.[59] The torque produced is a product of the force of a contraction times the distance the force is applied from the joint (lever arm). As the joint is moved through a range of motion, the resulting change in muscle length affects the length-tension of the muscle. Muscles are designed to work optimally from a predesigned position (line of pull). Altering joint positions, or line of pull, through postural abnormalities will alter the biomechanical efficiency of muscles. Furthermore, once muscles have adapted to their new and altered positions, an attempt by the therapist to change the positions will have an equally negative effect on function. Therapists must be aware of this and include rehabilitative exercises to avoid potential deleterious effects of posture re-education or quadrant balancing with shoe lifts.

Abnormalities in length, tension, or line of pull cause an abnormal demand on, or response from, the muscle. If this demand exceeds the mus-

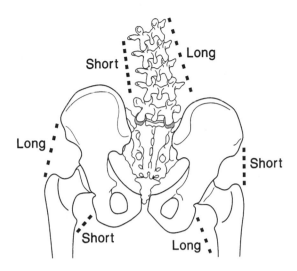

Figure 4-7 The effect of leg length asymmetry on muscle length. In response to postural asymmetries, muscles will structurally lengthen or shorten to adapt to their new position. (Courtesy of R Jackson, PT, OCS.)

cle's original design specifications, then inflammation and pain will result. Treatment directed to the tissue itself will be grossly inadequate. The painful tissue may need direct treatment, but this secondary treatment will be successful only if the primary cause of the overuse is eliminated. This brings us back to functional postural dynamics. That is the basis for understanding muscle biomechanics.

Principles of Movement

A finite amount of motion is necessary to walk, run, or execute our daily activities. These movements are predictable, but individual variations will occur. When a movement is lost in a joint, for whatever reason, the body will compensate at another joint or series of joints that are in phase with the affected joint.

A linkage system in the body is the framework that defines the mechanisms and interrelationships behind coordinated muscle activity.[17]

Joints are skeletal fulcrums and they are linked to one another by ligaments, capsules, and muscles. These motion units are connected in series to the spine. They must cooperate in function for the health and integrity of the whole. If acting in isolation, they will break down.

For instance, while a person is descending stairs, the knee must absorb more than 3.7 times the person's body weight. The knee cannot possibly tolerate this repetitive impact loading or it will break down. Therefore, the majority of the forces are transmitted proximal to the hip, pelvis, and spine and are dissipated or rechanneled into forward momentum.[17]

Joint motion that occurs in one plane is referred to as 1 degree of freedom of that joint. When moving through two or three planes, a joint is designated as having 2 or 3 degrees of freedom.

The lower extremity and trunk working together have 25 or more degrees of freedom. Limitation of joint range in the lower half may reduce the degrees of freedom normally available to the segments. If a typical functional task involving several segments is attempted, movement at the involved joint may not occur. Therefore, the other segments need to compensate, and the task will be carried out in an abnormal fashion.[65]

The inherently large number of degrees of freedom in the lower half minimizes the effects of a single joint dysfunction. In fact, dysfunction in the lower half is common and usually pain free. When looking at chronic pain, we must look at the total picture of dysfunction, which will help us to understand the sum total of abnormal forces acting on the affected tissue. This will help to direct treatment or the plan of correction.

The trunk must be considered the center of motion. A strong trunk aids in balance, coordination, and strength,[17,67,68] and, in fact, is the engine that drives locomotion.[67] Knott and Voss[69] stated that proximal muscle strength and coordination occur through four stages:

1. Mobility. Movement precedes posture—that is, mobility of the joints is needed to alter a position or to assume a posture.
2. Stability. Strength is needed to maintain a posture.
3. Controlled mobility, such as gait, requires distal stability and proximal mobility. This is why foot function is so important clinically. The foot is the body's articulation with the earth. If the foot is not stable, both structurally and functionally, then proximal function will be impaired. We will soon review numerous studies that show this to be true.
4. Skill. Fine motor skills and athletic performance require proximal stability and distal mobility. In the upper extremity, this relationship is obvious. In the lower extremity, distal mobility implies an open chain activity, such as kicking a ball. The proximal stability depends on stabilizing through the contralateral limb originating at the contralateral foot. Stability at the foot is critical.

Here again, we have come full circle. The body must have full *mobility* to maintain health. Normal functional mobility requires strong and stable proximal and distal segments. This is achieved through symmetric function, which allows muscles to function efficiently in the ways for which they were designed.

We know conclusively that back pain is best treated with exercise and restoration of functional mobility.[5,13,16,22–29] Back rehabilitation needs to be individually prescribed,[70] and that prescription needs to be based on the patient's specific needs. These needs are assessed only through a full evaluation of the lower half, both statically and dynamically. Too often the therapist or physician is looking only at the back, because this is where the pain is located. Back problems are often caused by lower extremity dysfunction. Dysfunction anywhere in the lower half can cause severe and chronic back pain.

Functional Relationships of the Lower Half

The body moves in predictable patterns.[69,71–73] What are the relationships between movement and LBP? The question arises about which motions, when restricted, could predispose an individual to chronic LBP. Is back pain caused by restricted motion of the lumbar spine or other areas as well? Is LBP caused by weakness of the trunk musculature?

Although there are some conflicts in the literature, we are fairly certain that trunk strength is a factor in patients who have chronic LBP. More specifically, trunk strength deficits strongly correlate with LBP.[70,74–77] Although there is really no agreement regarding the ratio of flexor-to-extensor strength in the LBP population,[70,76,77] there is no question that individuals who suffer from LBP have decreased trunk strength. These deficits can be on the magnitude of 40%.[75]

There are conflicts regarding the ability of a strong trunk to *prevent* the occurrence of LBP.[74,78] One might wonder how LBP is associated with weak trunk muscles, but strong trunk muscles do not necessarily prevent low back pain. If the cause is in the foot, then strong trunk musculature will not prevent the occurrence of LBP.

There is no question that pain inhibits muscle function, or muscle strength, in the area of pain. Therefore, it is reasonable to think that LBP will result in weak trunk musculature. The real question is, "What are the causes of LBP?" One of the factors that could cause LBP is weak trunk musculature. This is reasonable and is seen frequently by clinicians. In addition to weak trunk muscles, there are myriad causes of LBP. The problem can be in the foot, in gait, in the knee, in the hip, in the pelvis, and so forth.

Trunk and extremity mobility is frequently related to the development of LBP. An enormous amount of research has been done in this area.

If therapists were to choose one mechanical deficit that correlates most often with LBP, it would have to be tight hamstrings.[77,79–81] If nothing else, the therapist should stretch the hamstrings.

Actually, hypomobility throughout the lower limb correlates with an increased frequency of LBP,[18] especially in the hip joint. Hip joint motion restrictions have been directly linked to the development of chronic LBP.[79,80,82–88] Therefore, a clinician faced with a patient with chronic LBP must evaluate for and treat hip motion restrictions in the sagittal, frontal, and transverse planes.

The next area that should be examined is the spine itself. Does spinal hypomobility correlate with chronic low back pain? The research supports what we should know intuitively—lumbar range deficits are predictors of chronic LBP.[79–81,83,89–91] In fact, the problems with spinal hypomobility do not stop in the lumbar spine. Thoracolumbar mobility may be more significant in chronic LBP than lumbar mobility alone.[89]

What does all this research reveal? The human body is a machine. If therapists want the machine to work properly, they must make certain that all moving parts have freedom of motion. A mechanic who is working on a machine takes this for granted. Physical therapists should view the human machine the same way.

Common sense, coupled with research, confirms that there is a relationship between the hip, the pelvis, and the thoracolumbar spine. Therapists treating painful conditions in these regions must strive to restore strength and mobility.

Would it be reasonable to assume that the mobility and function of the joints farther down the chain might relate to the hip and spine? Could there be a functional relationship within all of the joints from the thoracic spine to the foot? Do each of the joints function as separate entities or do they cooperate as a single unit? There is evidence that the lower extremity joints cooperate as a single unit. Dysfunction in one joint can affect joints distant from the original site of injury.

Nicholas et al.[92] found that pathologic conditions of the foot and ankle caused weakness in hip abductors and adductors on the ipsilateral side. There were also nonsignificant trends in quadriceps and hamstring weakness. He concluded from these data that *the more distal the injury site, the greater the total weakness of the limb*. It is obvious that extremity joint injury causes strength and function problems distant to the site of the injury.

Closely related to this is the study by Jamarillo et al.[93] that demonstrated significant weakness of the hip joint musculature after knee surgery. They found all hip muscle groups weakened after knee surgery, especially hip extension.

A study by Matthews[94] related sacroiliac joint instability to development of osteoarthritis of the knee joint on the ipsilateral side. Stabilization of the hypermobile sacroiliac joint resulted in a decrease or resolution of knee pain.

Dananberg[95,96] suggested a direct causal relationship between functional hallux limitus (restriction during gait of the first metatarsophalangeal joint) and chronic postural pain. His studies showed that when functional hallux limitus was addressed in a select group of individuals with chronic LBP, 77% of these subjects showed improvements of 50–100% in their overall condition.

In a significant study on balance, Byl Nies and Sinnott[97] demonstrated conclusively that individuals with LBP have a disruption in their balance mechanism, poor one-footed balance, and a reliance on the hip-back mechanism rather than the foot-ankle mechanism to maintain balance. Remember, on the average, individuals must single-leg balance during gait 5,000 times each day. How do people with chronic back pain execute this? How does back pain influence balance during gait? Does the reliance on the hip-back mechanism to balance further perpetuate the LBP?

This study relates closely with a landmark study by Joanne Bullock-Saxton.[98] She compared two groups: an "injured" group who had previously sustained a severe unilateral ankle sprain, and a matched "control" group who had no previous lower limb injury. She studied changes in hip extension firing patterns and vibration perception. Her results were startling. There were changes in sensory perception (vibration) and hip extensor firing patterns with significant delays in gluteus maximus recruitment on the ipsilateral *and the contralateral sides*. These findings suggest that a reflex chain of events occurs after articular trauma, that altered sensation and abnormal muscular response can occur far from the site of the lesion, and that they are not even confined to the same side of the body. The work of Bennell and Goldie[99] dovetails nicely here. They found that application of ankle supports adversely affected the postural control system.

The research to date confirms that there is no such thing as a local joint injury. The lower half of the body is an integrated sensorimotor mechanism with all links in the system very much dependent on the other links for their ultimate efficiency of action. Obviously there is an integrated arthrokinetic reflex system working in the lower half that is integral in normal postural and movement patterns.

Nicholas and Marino[17] advised clinicians to appreciate the static and dynamic biomechanical and physiologic relationships that exist between the limbs and the trunk. Because all motions occur as a result of integrated cooperation of the individual segments, an isolated segment in dysfunction will affect the performance of the entire lower half.

The Challenge

The challenge of the lumbar spine analysis rests in the realization that pain in the lumbopelvic region comes from excessive forces, both structural and functional, entering the region. These forces may be generated locally or from a distant area of dysfunction. When examining the causes of low back pain, the therapist must consider all possibilities. The fact is, in most cases, we cannot clearly determine the exact cause of the pain. Following a comprehensive biomechanical evaluation, a therapist should develop a list of biomechanical deficits. Some problems may relate to strength, range, flexibility, gait, or posture. Which of these deficits are the actual cause of the patient's pain? It is usually impossible to tell. Treat all of the deficits and you have not only treated the present symptoms but future symptoms as well.

The role of the physical therapist is quite simple. We are movement specialists. Our job is to do a biomechanical assessment of the patient, the entire patient, both statically and dynamically. After the evaluation, the therapist should summarize the patient's deficits. After this, a plan is developed to treat the deficits and normalize function. When function is optimized, discharge follows. Discharge *is not* dependent on pain resolution. Discharge is dependent on maximal function biomechanically. We are, after all, mechanics of the body. When the system functions optimally, then the patient is discharged or referred on. Contrary to popular belief, pain is not our guide, and resolution of pain is not our primary goal. You will find that clinically, as mechanics are normalized, pain resolves.

References

1. Cavanaugh JM. Neural mechanisms of lumbar pain. Spine 1995;20:1804.
2. Garfin SR, Rydevik B, Lind B, Massie J. Spinal nerve root compression. Spine 1995;20:1810.
3. Saal JS. The role of inflammation in lumbar pain. Spine 1995;20:1821.
4. Hart LG, Deyo RA, Cherkin DC. Physician office visits for low back pain, frequency, clinical evaluation, and treatment patterns from a U.S. national survey. Spine 1995;20:11.
5. Battie MC, et al. Managing low back pain: attitudes and treatment preferences of physical therapists. Phys Ther 1994;74:219.

6. Schwarzer AC, et al. The relative contributions of the disc and zygapophyseal joint in chronic low back pain. Spine 1994;19:801.

7. Schwarzer AC, et al. The sacroiliac joint in chronic low back pain. Spine 1995;20:31.

8. Schwarzer AC. Clinical features of patients with pain stemming from the lumbar zygapophyseal joints—is the lumbar facet syndrome a clinical entity? Spine 1994;19:1132.

9. Waddell G. A new clinical model for the treatment of low-back pain. Spine 1987;12:632.

10. Porterfield J, DeRosa C. Mechanical Low Back Pain. Perspectives in Functional Anatomy. Philadelphia: WB Saunders, 1991.

11. Cornwall MW. Biomechanics of noncontractile tissue. Phys Ther 1984;64:1869.

12. Zairns B. Soft tissue injury and repair—biomechanical aspects. Int J Sports Med 1982;3:9.

13. Deyo R, et al. How many days of bed rest for acute low back pain? N Engl J Med 1986;315:1064.

14. Bullough P. Osteoarthritis: pathogenesis and aetiology. Br J Rheumatol 1984;23:166.

15. Goodfellow JW, Bullough PG. The pattern of aging of the articular cartilage of the elbow joint. J Bone Joint Surg Br 1967;49:175.

16. Mayer T, et al. Physical progress and residual impairment quantification after functional restoration, part I: lumbar mobility. Spine 1994;19:389.

17. Nicholas JA, Marino M. The relationship of injuries of the leg, foot, and ankle to proximal thigh strength in athletes. Foot Ankle Int 1987;7:218.

18. Fairbank JCT, et al. Influence of anthropometric factors and joint laxity in the incidence of adolescent back pain. Spine 1984;9:461.

19. Twomey LT. A rationale for the treatment of back pain and joint pain by manual therapy. Phys Ther 1992;72:885.

20. Jackson C, Brown M. Is there a role for exercise in the treatment of patients with low back pain? Clin Orthop Rel Res 1983;179:39.

21. Perry J. Anatomy and biomechanics of the hindfoot. Clin Orthop Rel Res 1983;177:9.

22. Gill C, et al. Low back pain: program description and outcome in a case series. J Orthop Sports Phys Ther 1994;20:11.

23. Alaranta H. Intensive physical and psychosocial training program for patients with chronic low back pain—a controlled clinical trial. Spine 1994;19:1339.

24. Nachemson A. Work for all. Clin Orthop Rel Res 1983;179:77.

25. Lankhorst G, et al. The natural history of idiopathic low back pain. A three-year follow-up study of spinal motion, pain, and functional capacity. Scand J Rehabil Med 1985;17:1.
26. Manniche C, et al. Intensive dynamic back exercises with or without hyperextension in chronic back pain after surgery for lumbar disc protrusion. Spine 1993;18:560.
27. Manniche C, et al. Clinical trial of postoperative dynamic back exercises after first lumbar discectomy. Spine 1993;18:92.
28. Timm K. A randomized-control study of active and passive treatments for chronic low back pain following L5 laminectomy. J Orthop Sports Phys Ther 1994;20(6):276.
29. Mitchell R, Carmen G. The functional restoration approach to the treatment of chronic pain in patients with soft tissue and back injuries. Spine 1994;19:633.
30. Radin E, et al. Role of mechanical factors in pathogenesis of primary osteoarthritis. Lancet 1972;March 4:519.
31. LeVeau B, Bernhardt D. Developmental biomechanics, effects of forces on the growth, development and maintenance of the human body. Phys Ther 1984;64:1874.
32. Lindgren U, Seireg A. The influence of mediolateral deformity, tibial torsion, and foot position on femorotibial load. Arch Orthop Trauma Surg 1989;108:22.
33. McCaw ST, Bates BT. Biomechanical implications of mild leg length inequality. Br J Sports Med 1991;25(1):10.
34. Radin EL, Burr DB, Caterson B, et al. Mechanical determinants of osteoarthrosis. Semin Arthritis Rheum 1991;21(3 Suppl 2):12.
35. Radin EL, Yang KH, Riegger C, et al. Relationship between lower limb dynamics and knee joint pain. J Orthop Res 1991;9:398.
36. Ting AJ, Tarr RR, Sarmiento A, et al. The role of subtalar motion and ankle contact pressure changes from angular deformities of the tibia. Foot Ankle Int 1987;7:290.
37. Ramsey PL, Hamilton W. Changes in tibiotalar area of contact caused by lateral talar shift. J Bone Joint Surg Am 1976;58:356.
38. Dixon A St. J, Campbell-Smith S. Long leg arthropathy. Ann Rheum Dis 1969;28:359.
39. Sicuranza B, et al. The short leg syndrome in obstetrics and gynecology. Am J Obstet Gynecol 1970;107:217.
40. Giles LGF, Taylor JR. Low-back pain associated with leg length inequality. Spine 1981;6:510.
41. Cummings G, et al. The effect of imposed leg length difference on pelvic bone symmetry. Spine 1993;18:368.

42. Schuit D, et al. Effect of heel lifts on ground reaction force patterns in subjects with structural leg length discrepancies. Phys Ther 1989; 69:663.

43. Subotnick S. Limb length discrepancies of the lower extremity (short leg syndrome). J Orthop Sports Phys Ther 1981;3:11.

44. Giles LGF, Taylor JR. Lumbar spine structural changes associated with leg length inequality. Spine 1982;7:159.

45. Gofton JP. Studies in osteoarthritis of the hip: part IV. Biomechanics and clinical consideration. Can Med Assoc J 1971;104:1007.

46. Cappozzo A. The forces and couples in the human trunk during level walking. Biomechanics 1983;16:265.

47. Enneking WF, Horowitz M. The intra-articular effects of immobilization on the human knee. J Bone Joint Surg Am 1972;54:973.

48. Kramer J. Pressure dependent fluid shifts in the intervertebral disc. Orthop Clin North Am 1977;8:211.

49. Farfan HF, et al. The effects of torsion on the lumbar intervertebral joints: the role of torsion in the production of disc degeneration. J Bone Joint Surg Am 1970;52:468.

50. Nachemson A. Towards a better understanding of low back pain: a review of the mechanics of the lumbar disc. Rheumatol Rehabil 1975;14:129.

51. Adams MA, Hutton WC. The effect of posture on the fluid content of lumbar intervertebral discs. Spine 1983;8:665.

52. Buckwalter JA. Aging and degeneration of the human intervertebral disc. Spine 1995;20:1307.

53. McNally DS, Adams MA, Goodship AE. Can intervertebral disc prolapse be predicted by disc mechanics? Spine 1993;18:1525.

54. Adams MA, Hutton WC. The effect of posture on the role of the apophysial joints in resisting intervertebral compressive forces. J Bone Joint Surg Br 1980;62:358.

55. Gotfried Y, et al. Facet joint changes after chemonucleolysis-induced disc space narrowing. Spine 1986;11:944.

56. Perennou D. Adult lumbar scoliosis. Spine 1994;19:123.

57. Friberg O. Clinical symptoms and biomechanics of lumbar spine and hip joint in leg length inequality. Spine 1983;8:643.

58. Gofton JP, Trueman GE. Studies in osteoarthritis of the hip: part II. Osteoarthritis of the hip and leg length disparity. Can Med Assoc J 1971;104:791.

59. Rab GT. Muscle. In J Rose, J Gamble (eds), Human Walking (2nd ed). Baltimore: Williams & Wilkins, 1994;109.

60. Korr I. Proprioceptors and somatic dysfunction. J Am Osteopath Assoc 1975;74:638.

61. Farfan HF. Form and function of the musculoskeletal system as revealed by mathematical analysis of the lumbar spine. Spine 1995;20:1462.
62. Guyton AC. Textbook of Medical Physiology. Philadelphia: WB Saunders, 1966;771.
63. Yekutiel M. The role of vertebral movement in gait: implications for manual therapy. J Man Manip Ther 1994;2:22.
64. Mueller MJ, et al. Differences in the gait characteristics of patients with diabetes and peripheral neuropathy compared with age-matched controls. Phys Ther 1994;74:299.
65. Deusinger R. Biomechanics in clinical practice. Phys Ther 1984; 64:1860.
66. Cerny K. Pathomechanics of stance, clinical concepts for analysis. Phys Ther 1984;64:1851.
67. Gracovetsky S. The Spinal Engine. New York: Springer-Verlag, 1988;286.
68. Voss D. Proprioceptive neuromuscular facilitation. Am J Phys Med 1967;46:838.
69. Knott M, Voss DE. Proprioceptive Neuromuscular Facilitation, Patterns and Techniques (2nd ed). New York: Harper & Row, 1968;111.
70. Pope MH, et al. The relationship between anthropometric, postural muscular, and mobility characteristics of males ages 18–55. Spine 1985;10:644.
71. Miller D, Morrison W. Prediction of segmental parameters using the hanavan human body model. Med Sci Sports 1975;7:207.
72. Miller D. Body segment contributions to sport skill performance: two contrasting approaches. Res Q Exercise Sport 1983;51:219.
73. Nicholas JA, et al. The importance of a simplified classification of motion in sports in relation to performance. Orthop Clin North Am 1977;8:499.
74. Biering-Sorenson F. Physical measurements as risk indicators for low-back trouble over a one-year period. Spine 1984;9:106.
75. McNeil T, et al. Trunk strengths in attempting flexion, extension, and lateral bending in healthy subjects and patients with low back disorders. Spine 1980;5:529.
76. Suzuki N, Endo S. A quantitative study of trunk muscle strength and fatigability in the low-back pain syndrome. Spine 1983;8:69.
77. Alston W, et al. A quantitative study of muscle factors in the chronic low back syndrome. J Am Geriatr Soc 1966;14:1041.
78. Nachemson A, Lindh M. Measurement of abdominal and back muscle strength with and without low back pain. Scand J Rehabil Med 1969;1:60.
79. Mellin G. Correlations of hip mobility with degree of back pain and lumbar spinal mobility in chronic low-back pain patients. Spine 1988;13:668.

80. Mellin G. Chronic low back pain in men 54–63 years of age-correlations of physical measurements with the degree of trouble and progress after treatment. Spine 1986;11:421.
81. Gajdosik R, et al. Influence of hamstring length on the standing position and flexion range of motion of the pelvic angle, lumbar angle and thoracic angle. J Orthop Sports Phys Ther 1994;20:213.
82. Mellin G. Decreased joint and spinal mobility associated with low back pain in young adults. J Spinal Disord 1990;3:238.
83. Mellin G, et al. A controlled study on the outcome of inpatient and outpatient treatment of low-back pain, part II. Scand J Rehabil Med 1989;21:91.
84. Ellison JB, et al. Patterns of hip rotation range of motion: a comparison between healthy subjects and patients with low back pain. Phys Ther 1990;70:537.
85. Nachemson A. Electromyographic studies on the vertebral portion of the psoas muscle. Acta Orthopedic Scand 1966;37:177.
86. Nachemson A. The possible importance of the psoas muscle for stabilization of the lumbar spine. Acta Orthopedic Scand 1968;39:47.
87. Offierski CM, MacNab MB. Hip-spine syndrome. Spine 1983;8:316.
88. Gracovetsky S, et al. The mechanism of the lumbar spine. Spine 1981;6:249.
89. Mellin G. Correlations of spinal mobility with degree of chronic low-back pain after correction for age and anthropometric factors. Spine 1987;12:464.
90. Hansson T, et al. The bone mineral content of the lumbar spine in patients with chronic low-back pain. Spine 1985;10:158.
91. Farfan HF. The biomechanical advantage of lordosis and hip extension for upright activity—man as compared with other anthropods. Spine 1978;3:336.
92. Nicholas J, et al. A study of thigh muscle weakness in different pathological states of the lower extremity. Am J Sports Med 1976;4:241.
93. Jamarillo J, et al. Hip isometric strength following knee surgery. J Orthop Sports Phys Ther 1994;20:160.
94. Matthews JH. A new approach to the treatment of osteoarthritis of the knee: prolotherapy of the ipsilateral sacroiliac ligaments. J Orthop Med 1995;17(3):101.
95. Dananberg HJ. Gait style as an etiology to chronic postural pain, part I, functional hallux limitus. J Am Podiatr Med Assoc 1993;83:433.
96. Dananberg HJ. Gait style as an etiology to chronic postural pain, part II, postural compensatory process. J Am Podiatr Med Assoc 1993;83:615.

97. Byl Nies N, Sinnott PL. Variations in balance and body sway in middle-aged adults, subjects with healthy backs compared with subjects with low-back dysfunction. Spine 1991;16:325.
98. Bullock-Saxton JE. Local sensation changes and altered hip muscle function following severe ankle sprain. Phys Ther 1994;74:17.
99. Bennell K, Goldie P. The differential effects of external ankle support on postural control. J Orthop Sports Phys Ther 1994;20:287.

III

Management

5

Patient Management
Brian P. D'Orazio

In the classic biomedical model of pain, pathologic condition determines treatment. Identification of pathologic entities among people with low back pain (LBP), however, has been an elusive task, leading Nachemson to conclude that most patients with LBP have no identifiable pathologic condition.[1] Equally problematic is the often poor correlation between identifiable pathologic entities and symptoms. As an example, degenerative changes in the lumbar spine are common; however, these changes exist in the population both with and without LBP. The Quebec Task Force reported in Chapter 3 of its monograph, "it is generally impossible to corroborate clinical observations through histologic studies because, on one hand, the usual benignity of spinal disorders does not justify that tissue be removed and, on the other, there is often no modification of tissue identifiable through current methods."[2] Videman reported that, "back pain is basically a complaint not an illness."[3]

De Rosa offered that treatment often is a combination of the clinician's bias about which tissues are responsible for LBP in combination with the amount of distress the patient projects about the condition. Thus, intervention is often the result of "treatment approaches in search of a syndrome."[4]

If treatment cannot be based on a 1 to 1 correlation between pathologic condition and symptoms, then perhaps La Rocca's editorial comments help focus the issue: "The problem emanates from the lack of a comprehensive and unifying problem-solving strategy to appraise the relevant data and from them to establish policy and procedures for implementing effective management while remaining receptive to new learning."[5] D'Orazio reported, "accepting that a solid diagnosis is often impossible, with many diagnoses being verified retrospectively, then the term diagnosis should most often be replaced by the term hypothesis and treatment should proceed using clinical algorithms."[6] Because physical and psychosocial variables are commonly

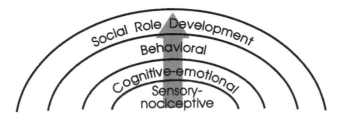

Figure 5-1 Developmental sequence of chronic pain development. (Reprinted with permission from TC Toomey. Psychological Assessment Strategies for Low Back Pain Patients in the Physical Therapy Setting. In BP D'Orazio [ed], Back Pain Rehabilitation. Boston: Andover Medical Publishers, 1993;91.)

concurrent issues, the development of a clinical algorithm for patient management must consider known variables that can act as barriers to recovery. The remainder of this chapter focuses principally on psychosocial issues that can act as barriers to recovery.

Low Back Pain: A Multifactorial Problem

Expression of Pain

Pain is a multifactorial experience occasionally demanding a multidisciplinary approach to its management. Classic pain models rely on symptom expression to be an accurate predictor of tissue damage. Applying this model to all patients will lead to inappropriate management, because the expression of pain is influenced by many factors. If viewed developmentally, "the meaning of pain tends to vary along a temporal dimension from a sensory signal of nociception to an increasingly unified sequence of emotions, cognitions, behaviors and social roles."[7] Figure 5-1 depicts a theoretical model for sequential behavioral development among chronic pain patients. Patients will not necessarily progress through all dimensions of this model.

Temporal Dimensions of Pain

Temporal factors become especially important when the expected time frame of recovery and the patient's actual rate of recovery are significantly different. Most of the literature agrees that LBP persisting beyond 6 months meets the definition of chronic. The Quebec Task Force defined chronic pain as pain existing longer than 7 weeks, whereas the subacute phase was defined as 7 days to 7 weeks, a time frame during which normal healing can be expected. This is presumed to be true even when a specific pathologic condition cannot be identified. The acute phase is reserved for pain present during the first 7 days.[2]

Delitto and colleagues offered that temporal categories of acute, subacute, and chronic pain are often arbitrary and lack meaning when establishing a plan of care.[8] Clearly, specific time frames are not the only variable to be considered; however, time is a significant variable. As time passes, iatrogenic changes take place that can serve ultimately to compromise the final outcome. If joints are not moved on a regular basis, it is well understood that articular cartilage is damaged. Furthermore, connective tissue bonds are formed to replace muscle tissue, and flexibility is lost. If enough time passes, the central nervous system also changes. This critical temporal dimension of pain is highlighted by La Rocca's comments: "Further, modern algology has identified distinct differences between acute and chronic pain, in which the latter is not merely a continuation of the former over time. Instead, a host of organic changes occur in the neuraxis in response to nociception that perpetuates pain independent of psychosocial considerations."[5] Whatever the reason, a patient with protracted pain is less likely to experience a complete resolution of symptoms. In patients with work-related injuries to the low back, 74.2% return to work within 4 weeks. This contrasts with 7.4% of workers who remain out of work for more than 6 months and account for 75.6% of the compensatory costs for their injuries[2] (Figure 5-2). Delitto's argument notwithstanding, many decision-making processes for this chapter will be time-based.

This chapter's management time frames are based mostly on the Quebec Task Force's recommendations, which consider both normal healing rates as well as known percentages of recovery. Consequently, the management time frames will be divided into acute, subacute, prechronic, and chronic (Table 5-1).[2]

The term *prechronic* is intended to bridge the gap between subacute and chronic and serves as a warning for clinicians to aggressively manage the patient's complaints. Data from Waddell indicate that only 50% of patients return to their prior work state if they were injured at work and have been out of work for more than 6 months. After 2 years, virtually none of the patients ever return to gainful employment.[9] For patients who enter multidisciplinary programs, the statistics vary on the percentage that ultimately return to work; however, excellent results have been obtained by this method, with between 50% and 80% of those patients returning to some type of employment.[10–13] Hazard et al. reported that among chronic back pain patients in their study, 81% of the program graduates returned to work

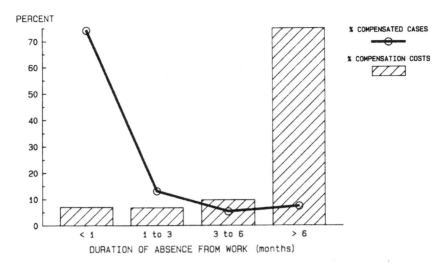

Figure 5-2 Compensation costs for back injury by duration of absence from work. (Reprinted with permission from WO Spitzer, FE LeBlanc, M Dupuis, et al. Scientific approach to the assessment and management of activity related spinal disorders: a monograph for clinicians. Report of the Quebec Task Force on Spinal Disorders. Spine 1987;12[Suppl 7]:S15.)

Table 5-1 Temporal Classification of Symptom Duration

Management classification	Duration of symptoms
Acute	0–7 days
Subacute	7 days–7 weeks
Prechronic	7 weeks–6 months
Chronic	Longer than 6 months

Source: Adapted with permission from WO Spitzer, FE LeBlanc, M Dupuis, et al. Scientific approach to the assessment and management of activity related spinal disorders: a monograph for clinicians. Report of the Quebec Task Force on Spinal Disorders. Spine 1987;12(Suppl 7):S16.

compared with 40% of those who dropped out of the program and 29% of those who were denied admission to the program by the insurance company.[11] The study by Mayer et al. demonstrated similar results.[13] These statistics support the need for a structured multidisciplinary approach for patients who have chronic pain.

Recognizing Barriers to Recovery

Defining the Barriers

Barriers to recovery are those events or circumstances that impede the patient's functional recovery. During the initial evaluation and early in treatment, the clinician must identify barriers that may delay or prevent recovery. Some of these barriers preclude initiating treatment.

Delitto's contention is that the severity of disability is more useful than the time from injury as a guide to patient classification and management.[8] This approach could be viewed as biobehavioral. Feurstein and Beattie described biobehavioral factors as "a set of psychological, environmental and psychophysiological processes that attenuate or exacerbate the discrepancy among pathology, pain, impairment, functional limitation and disabilities."[14] These factors can predate an injury, creating barriers to recovery.[15] Barriers to recovery may emerge during treatment, highlighting the necessity for ongoing interactions with the patient. The identification of barriers to recovery early in treatment, preferably during the examination, should cause the clinician to initiate some preliminary multidisciplinary efforts in order to reduce the probability of an acutely injured individual's symptoms becoming chronic. A summary of barriers to recovery is included in Table 5-2. Most of these are self-explanatory, but a few warrant further explanation and are discussed in the next section of this chapter.

Management of Specific Barriers

Once specific barriers to recovery have been identified, management can proceed in a logical manner but will require skill and an appropriate knowledge base. The beginning of all management strategies is the assertion that the patient's pain is real. It is important to openly acknowledge this to the patient in order to gain his or her confidence. Meilman believes that "[i]f there is any doubt in the physical therapist's mind, this will be communicated wittingly or unwittingly to the patient and the patient will either become uncooperative or will go to great lengths to prove that the pain is real. Remember that the patient's credibility has likely been questioned already by treating physicians, friends, family members and employers. Further questioning will serve only to alienate the clinician from the patient and may make the patient more difficult, if not impossible, to reach. In treatment, it is always important to accept the pain as real and never to question it."[16] The number of patients who knowingly are exaggerating their complaint are few, despite beliefs to the contrary by society at large and insurance companies in particular.

Table 5-2 Barriers to Recovery

 1. Poor match of worker to task

 2. Low educational background

 3. History of problems on the job

 4. Depression

 5. Symptom magnification

 6. Secondary gain

 7. Illness

 8. Smoking

 9. Substance abuse

10. History of being abused as a child

11. Past failures with treatment

12. Financial constraints

13. Difficulties with transportation

14. Abnormal fear of reinjury

15. Overly protective spouse

16. Clinicians who warn against painful activity

17. Sick role familiarity

18. Anxiety

19. Fear of discrimination from work

20. Fear of dismissal from work

21. Poor understanding of the reasons for treatment

22. Conflicting information regarding pathology

23. Anxious about degenerative changes

24. Anxiety about remaining pathology in adjacent motion segments after surgery

Depression

Patients who exhibit four or more of the following nine symptoms continually for more than 2 weeks may be experiencing a major depressive episode: depressed mood, loss of interest in activities, insomnia, oversleeping or early morning waking, decreased energy, significant weight gain or loss, feelings of hopelessness, inability to concentrate, recurrent thoughts of death or suicide, and restlessness. According to the *Johns Hopkins White Papers*, in addition to disturbances in thinking, patients may also have abnormalities in body function, such as decreased sexual drive, constipation, or weight loss.[17] Not all depressions require psychological intervention. Many depressions are situational and resolve as the physical symptoms resolve. If physical signs are improving but the patient's mood remains depressed, seek further help from a mental health professional. If the patient answers affirmative to suicidal ideation (item 9 on the Beck's Depression Inventory), seek immediate referral to a mental health professional.

Secondary Gain

Issues of secondary gain are problematic. Patients are not usually forthcoming in discussing a possible financial reward to their disability. Conversely, clinicians are commonly aware of financial hardships. Secondary gain must be suspected as an issue if an attorney has been retained and if the patient's income on workers' compensation is close to or exceeds his or her working income. If the clinician suspects secondary gain is an issue, a case manager should be involved. If attempts to focus on function in treatment are unsuccessful, the clinician should refer to Chapter 6 for specific therapeutic exercise approaches for this category of patient.

Past Treatment Failures

A common barrier to recovery is past failures with treatment. Feurstein and Beattie[14] offered that patients with failed attempts at treatment may feel "that function cannot be restored until a cause for the pain is identified and eliminated." The authors further stated that "the cyclical nature of the process makes it very difficult for the clinician to intervene, particularly if a belief system is not identified and addressed."[14] Any time a patient has previously been treated without success, full details of the patient's previous treatment regimen should be obtained and thoroughly reviewed. Treatment that did not facilitate functional goals or positively change signs and symptoms must be identified and eliminated. In the first several treatment sessions, repetitions of each exercise may need to be increased by only one repetition per set, allowing the patient to see a daily progression without exacerbation of symptoms. As the patient gains confidence, he or she will be more fully invested in the program and reasonable increases in exercise levels can be initiated. Treatment is similar for patients who are abnormally anxious about their condition or abnormally fear reinjury.

Fear of Reinjury

Patients with an abnormal fear of reinjury or who are overly anxious about symptoms will be slow to respond to therapeutic intervention until consistent successes with treatment have been achieved. It is helpful to quickly return the patient to light duty work. Often, this solves the problem. Extensive documentation of both treatment and responses is necessary, as is aggressive discharge planning. Diagnostic tests that reassure the patient are essential. Those administering the test must be cautioned to offer no information to the patient. Discussion of diagnostic tests is the responsibility of the primary treating clinician.

Malingering

Unfortunately, the term *symptom magnification* (SM) has become synonymous with malingering. As Meilman reported, "most professionals working in the field agree that malingering is an extremely rare phenomenon. A good working assumption is that patients are accurately representing their experience unless there is convincing evidence to the contrary—for example, a patient who cannot walk in the office but is observed walking on the street and is known to make more money on disability than when last employed."[16] If the clinician observes the patient to be engaging in clearly fraudulent activity, such as directly observing the patient walking normally in the community when in the office the patient is barely ambulatory with a cane, every attempt should be made to terminate treatment at the earliest possible time. Decisions regarding this patient should be made only after consultation with all parties involved. If the patient has filed a workers' compensation claim or is suing for an out-of-work accident, legal action against the patient may be initiated by the insurance company.

A conscious desire to fake an injury is only one of a multitude of explanations for displays of nonorganic pain behaviors. It is tempting to conclude that a patient is malingering. The insurance companies have a vested interest in discontinuing treatment and salary payment for a person who is injured on the job. Consequently, this conflict of interest in combination with much publicized fraudulent schemes by patients greatly influences the insurance carrier's viewpoint. Furthermore, it is embarrassing to invest in a patient's treatment and later find out the patient's presentation of symptoms was fraudulent. Nevertheless, labeling a patient as a malingerer has tremendous legal and social consequences. If you believe the patient is malingering, seek another opinion, if possible from someone in the mental health field.

Nonorganic Pain Behaviors

Nonorganic pain behaviors are directly observable and testable behaviors indicating nonorganic pathologic conditions (Table 5-3). Frequently the result of several barriers to recovery, "[p]ain behaviors," Meilman

Table 5-3 Nonorganic Pain Behaviors

1. Use of supportive devices
2. Excessive amount of recumbent time secondary to pain
3. Excessive grimacing with activities that do not involve the low back
4. Frequently rubbing the area of pain
5. Frequent verbal descriptions of pain
6. Excessive dependency on family and health care providers
7. Meandering
8. Limping in the absence of an identifiable physiologic reason
9. Moaning
10. Frequently saying "I can't" when asked to perform simple activities

Source: Adapted from G Waddell, JA McCulloch, E Kummel, et al. Nonorganic physical signs in low back pain. Spine 1979;5:117.

stated, "keep the patient focused on the pain and perpetuate the disability. Effective chronic pain management entails helping patients identify their pain behaviors and then working with them to eliminate these forms of communication."[16]

Many of these behaviors are extinguished once the clinician reassures the patient that he or she accepts the patient's pain complaint as real and indicates that every effort will be made to speed the patient's recovery. Under most circumstances, pain behaviors abate as function improves. If this does not occur, further psychosocial screening should be performed and other health professionals involved in the patient's case should be consulted.

Many of the nonorganic pain behaviors will be eliminated as the patient gains confidence in the clinician. For example, if the patient unnecessarily uses a cane for ambulation, it could be suggested after the first 2 weeks of treatment that the patient has improved enough that the cane is no longer required while in the office. Later, the suggestion could be advanced that the cane be eliminated for all activities. If the patient uses excessive grimacing or gesturing during activities, the clinician can extinguish these behaviors by asking the patient to verbalize what is being experienced. The clinician must then acknowledge the patient's pain but offer that the assigned task will be easier with repetition. The physical therapist should continue to reinforce verbalization rather than excessive grimacing or gesturing as a means to express pain.

Multiple nonorganic pain behaviors, including testable behaviors during an examination, are collectively referred to as *SM*. Matheson defined SM as

Table 5-4 Waddell's Nonorganic Physical Signs Worksheet

Physical signs	Result
1. Simulation	+ or −
a. Axial loading	
b. Simulated trunk rotation	
2. Regional	+ or −
a. Nonanatomic sensory dermatome	
b. Nonanatomic motor myotome	
3. Tenderness	+ or −
a. Light pinching	
b. Superficial palpation	
4. Overreaction during physical examination	+ or −
5. Distracted straight leg raise	+ or −
a. Sitting versus recumbent	

Note: Abnormal illness behaviors are present when the clinician finds at least three out of five "positive." If one part of the physical sign being tested is abnormal, then the entire section is considered positive.
Source: Adapted from Waddell G, McCulloch JA, Kummel E, et al. Nonorganic physical signs in low back pain. Spine 1979;5:117.

"a conscious or unconscious self destructive, socially reinforced behavioral response pattern consisting of reports or displays of symptoms that function to control the life circumstances of the sufferer."[18] King simplified this definition by stating, "the patient's response, or disability, is much greater than expected based on the objective findings."[19] Waddell described specific SM tests that have become standards in the physical examination of patients with LBP (Table 5-4).[20]

As indicated previously, nonorganic pain behaviors are frequently the result of specific barriers to recovery. Table 5-5 details specific biobehavioral factors that act as barriers to recovery, many of which have been alluded to previously.

Patient Management

What Are the Goals?

There are two primary sets of treatment goals: yours and the patient's. The extent to which these are congruent will define the amount of patient education required.

Table 5-5 Biobehavioral Factors that May Generate Nonorganic Pain Behaviors

Barrier	Manifestation of the barrier
Disease conviction (the belief that pain is a sign of major health problems)	Increased distress leading to anxiety and fear Decreased pain tolerance The patient searches for a "correct" diagnosis The patient believes that function cannot be restored before the underlying cause of his or her pain is found and cured
Cognitive-perceptual bias (interpreting physical symptoms or associated emotional distress as a sign of illness)	Exaggerated pain response with movement or gentle touch High levels of anxiety
Perceived illness (the belief of the patient that he or she is too disabled to perform a specific task despite little objective evidence of impairment)	Fear of reinjury Avoidance of negative consequences Anxiety, depression, or both
Fear of pain (the fear of pain creates a reaction before the actual sensation of pain)	Muscle guarding Reduction in activity
Perceptions of work and family (perceptions characterized by low job satisfaction, limited supervisory support, lack of job clarity, and support at home for the sick role)	Exacerbations of low back pain Maintenance of low back pain Prolonged disability in the absence of proportionate impairment

Source: Adapted from M Feurstein, P Beattie. Biobehavioral factors affecting pain and disability and low back pain: mechanics and assessment. Phys Ther 1995;75:267.

A common patient goal is to become pain free. Although this is an understandable goal, it is not always realistic. For chronic pain patients, this is always considered a negative goal because the focus is on pain, not function. The challenge is to assist patients in refocusing their attention on function. This is especially difficult for patients with a disease conviction, believing the underlying pathologic condition remains undiscovered.

Another negative goal is the desire to start a business or change jobs. This is considered a negative goal because the clinical focus on function may be in conflict with the patient's motivation. In some instances, the patient will use the circumstances of the injury to allow for the time and finances necessary to start a business or change jobs.

Another common goal is returning to work or some specific activity that the patient has been avoiding because of LBP. This goal is usually congruent with the clinician's primary goal of helping the patient regain his or her preinjury level of function. An on-site visit to the patient's workplace or a functional capacities examination may help define the therapeutic course required to achieve this goal. As noted in Table 5-2, a poor match of the worker to the task is a significant barrier.

The patient is often overwhelmed by the many activities that have been taken away by LBP. Often, activity modification allows the patient to immediately resume some activities, thereby lessening the psychosocial burden. Additionally, the increased activity level is often beneficial. Specific modifications are available in many self-help guides.

Once the patient's goals are discussed, the clinician must formulate reasonable treatment goals. The clinician should make a list of functional outcomes that are anticipated within a 2- to 3-week time frame from treatment and then by the end of treatment. These likely will include functional tasks with specific variables for walking distances, sitting time, standing time, and weight-lifting limits from various heights.

Although functional goals are necessary, resolution of specific impairments or dysfunctions must also be goals to limit future trauma and dysfunction. The treatment of impairment was discussed in previous chapters.

Goals for Management

In Chapter 5 of the report by the Quebec Task Force on Spinal Disorders, the authors wrote "management strategies should be directed at maximizing the number of workers returning to work before one month and minimizing the numbers whose spinal disorder keeps them idle for longer than six months. Thus, returning to work as a management objective is both sound clinically and economically."[2] The authors further summarized their management goals as "(1) [e]arly recognition of individuals who fall into the chronic pain syndrome category; (2) [a]ssurance of validity and consistency in diagnosis; (3) [e]arly coordination in the management of the condition with specialists in the areas of spinal disorders, pain and work rehabilitation; [and] (4) [d]elivery of consistent reassurance to the worker throughout the condition."[2] Hazard offered that treatment should continue to proceed as long as progress is being made and until maximum medical improvement has been achieved. The iatrogenic changes that take place with spinal injuries can be substantial and, in combination with psychosocial ramifications, premature termination of treatment will likely lead to increased economic cost and disability.[11]

Once the barriers to the patient's recovery are identified, strategies for management should be reviewed. If the patient demonstrates early signs of barriers to recovery that will likely have a negative impact later, it is much better to manage those problems early in treatment. In my office, a pain management director with a master's degree in psychology works with patients as a case manager, motivator, psychosocial screener, and general troubleshooter. This has made a tremendous difference in patient care. Psychosocial concerns cannot be ignored; in fact, they have proved to be the most consistent and reliable predictor of outcomes. Attempting to treat all cases of LBP without the help of a case worker or mental health professional will be frustrating for the clinician and for the patient.[21–23]

An Algorithm for Low Back Pain Management

Figure 5-3A is a temporal patient management algorithm that offers management suggestions based on common presentations of patients injured in the workplace. This algorithm could easily be adapted to non-workplace injuries because the decision-making process is unchanged.

In the acute injury phase, there are very few circumstances that require consultation with a case manager or mental health care professional. Measures should be taken to rule out disease or neurologic involvement, to develop a working diagnosis, and to initiate conservative care appropriate to the extent of the injury. By collecting information on the patient's work duties, the return-to-work process has already been initiated. For those with chronic LBP, all patients need to be referred for a multidisciplinary team evaluation, because the condition clearly falls outside the normal areas of histologic healing.

As identified in Figure 5-3A, acute pain patients are usually exempt from a referral to a multidisciplinary program. An exception is a former chronic pain patient who has suffered a recent exacerbation of the condition and at the initial evaluation is already demonstrating signs of anxiety or other barriers. A multidisciplinary team approach to this patient's care should be initiated immediately.

Figure 5-3B is an algorithm for the subacute patient. If the patient is progressing as anticipated, a return to light-duty work, if appropriate, helps reduce anxieties about returning to work. The patient should not be placed in a light-duty job that is inappropriate or that could delay progression of that patient's conservative care.

Before the end of 7 weeks, most patients should return to normal work and daily activities. Early identification of patients who are not progressing as anticipated helps identify specific barriers to recovery that may be slowing the patient's progress or that could serve to lead the patient into a chronic pain syndrome. In this algorithm, SMS stands for symptom magnification syndrome.

If the patient is not progressing as anticipated, conferring with a case management worker or mental health professional may be necessary. Patients should be evaluated for barriers to recovery and possible SMS. When neither are found, the patient should be re-evaluated, the treatment

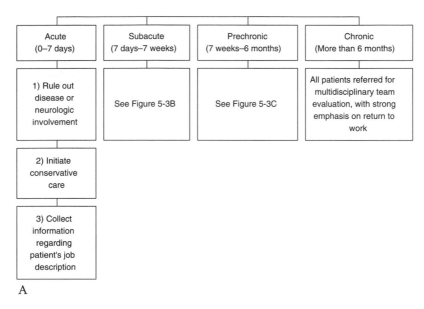

A

Figure 5-3 (A) Patient management algorithm. (B) Subacute pain (7 days to 7 weeks). (C) Prechronic pain (7 weeks to 6 months). (SMS = symptom magnification syndrome; MRI = magnetic resonance imaging; EMG = electromyography; FCE = functional capacities evaluation.)

program adjusted, and another practitioner consulted if the reason for the limited progress is not clear.

If the barriers to recovery are not significant but SMS is present, a mental health professional should be consulted and treatment that emphasizes behavioral modification and function should be initiated. Insignificant barriers are those that can be managed through either education or short-term treatment. An example is a patient who does not understand why he or she is being treated. Another example would be conflicting information about the patient's pathologic condition. This can usually be solved with a meeting between clinicians followed by a meeting with the patient. Another insignificant barrier could be transportation, which often can be solved with a call to the rehabilitation nurse or the case adjuster.

Many potential barriers to recovery are listed in Table 5-2. Significant barriers represent those that cannot be easily solved. Barriers such as depression, illness, secondary gain, and substance abuse, present greater challenges. For a patient with significant barriers and SMS, referral to a multidisciplinary team for evaluation and treatment is indicated.

Figure 5-3C details management guidelines for prechronic patients. As stated previously, this classification is a bridge between subacute and chronic. At this stage, the patient must be aggressively managed to prevent

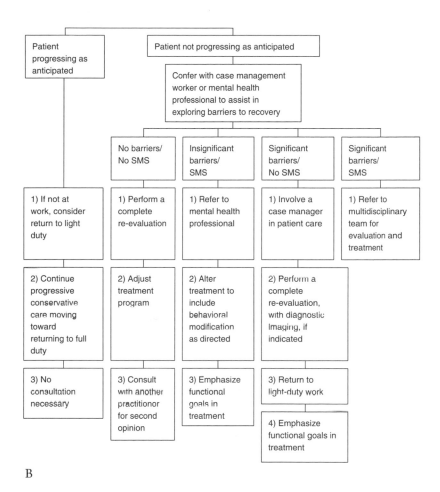

Patient progressing as anticipated	Patient not progressing as anticipated			
	Confer with case management worker or mental health professional to assist in exploring barriers to recovery			
	No barriers/ No SMS	Insignificant barriers/ SMS	Significant barriers/ No SMS	Significant barriers/ SMS
1) If not at work, consider return to light duty	1) Perform a complete re-evaluation	1) Refer to mental health professional	1) Involve a case manager in patient care	1) Refer to multidisciplinary team for evaluation and treatment
2) Continue progressive conservative care moving toward returning to full duty	2) Adjust treatment program	2) Alter treatment to include behavioral modification as directed	2) Perform a complete re-evaluation, with diagnostic imaging, if indicated	
3) No consultation necessary	3) Consult with another practitioner for second opinion	3) Emphasize functional goals in treatment	3) Return to light-duty work	
			4) Emphasize functional goals in treatment	

B

the condition from becoming chronic. The first category, as with Figure 5-3B, concerns the patient who is progressing as anticipated. At this stage, the patient usually is well advanced in rehabilitation and probably has the ability to return to some form of work. The health care provider, especially the physical therapist, should be cognizant that most patients are able to return to full-duty work within 4 weeks after an injury.

The process for evaluating prechronic and subacute LBP patients is the same. The emphasis is slightly different in that after 7 weeks a stronger emphasis is placed on returning the patient to some level of employment. Even if the patient is progressing as anticipated, a functional capacities evaluation should be performed for appropriate placement of the patient at his or her previous place of employment. If the patient is not progressing as anticipated, the four categories for possible reasons remain unchanged. A case manager or mental health professional can be helpful in exploring pos-

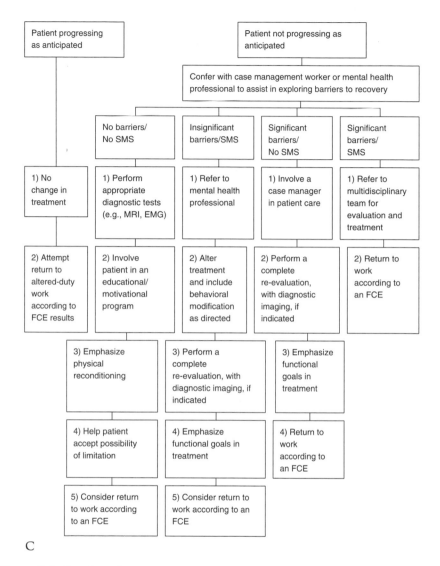

C

Figure 5-3 *Continued*

sible reasons for limited progress. In the first category, where the patient has no barriers to returning to work and there is no evidence of SMS, it would be appropriate to perform a functional capacities evaluation if diagnostic testing and re-examination failed to produce evidence of a reason why the patient should not return to work at some level. This is also true for category 2, insignificant barriers/SMS, depending on the recommendations of the mental health professional. In the last two categories, a functional capacities evaluation should be performed routinely with a strong emphasis on immediately returning the patient to some level of employment.

Conclusion

Patient management is perhaps the most overlooked facet of treatment for patients with LBP. The accumulation of multiple technical treatment strategies for LBP patients is not enough. The specific management pathways outlined in Figure 5-3 should help the clinician avoid the pitfalls of attempting treatment on patients who require specialized management skills.

If management of LBP patients is the most overlooked facet of care, the infrequent referral of LBP patients to specific programs or clinicians who possess appropriate management skills for that level of patient is testimony to an unwillingness to recognize our clinical limitations. Unfortunately, this failing is common among physical therapists and desperately needs to be corrected in academic and clinical centers.

References

1. Nachemson AL. Newest knowledge of low back pain: a critical look. Clin Orthop 1992;279:8.
2. Spitzer WO, LeBlanc FE, Dupuis M, et al. Scientific approach to the assessment and management of activity-related spinal disorders: a monograph for clinicians. Report of the Quebec Task Force on spinal disorders. Spine 1987;12(Suppl 7):S9.
3. Videman T. Evaluation of the prevention of occupational low-back pain. Spine 1991;16:685.
4. De Rosa CP. Invited commentaries. In: Delitto A, Erhard RE, Bowling RW. A treatment-based classification approach to low back syndrome: identifying and staging patients for conservative treatment. Phys Ther 1995;75:485.
5. La Rocca H. Editorial. In WO Spitzer, FE LeBlanc, M Dupuis (eds), et al. Scientific approach to the assessment and management of activity-related spinal disorders: a monograph for clinicians. Report of the Quebec Task Force on Spinal Disorders. Spine 1987;12(Suppl 7):S8.
6. D'Orazio BP. Introduction. In BP D'Orazio (ed), Back Pain Rehabilitation. Boston: Andover Medical Publishers, 1993;xx.
7. Toomey TC. Psychological Assessment Strategies for Low-Back Pain Patients in the Physical Therapy Setting. In BP D'Orazio (ed), Back Pain Rehabilitation. Boston: Andover Medical Publishers, 1993;87.

8. Delitto A, Erhard RE, Bowling RW. A treatment-based classification approach to low back syndrome: identifying and staging patients for conservative treatment. Phys Ther 1995;75:470.

9. Waddell G. A new clinical model for the treatment of low-back pain. Spine 1987;12:632.

10. Werneke MW, Harris DE, Lichter RL. Clinical effectiveness of behavioral signs for screening chronic low-back pain after surgery for lumbar disc protrusion: a clinical trial. Spine 1993;18:2412.

11. Hazard RG, Fenwick JW, Kalisch SM, et al. Functional restoration with behavioral support: a one-year prospective study of patients with chronic low-back pain. Spine 1991;16:615.

12. Cats-Baril WL, Frymoyer JW. Demographic factors associated with the prevalence of disability in the general population: analysis of the NHANAE I database. Spine 1991;16:671.

13. Mayer TG, Gatchel RJ, Kishino N, et al. Objective assessment of spine function following industrial injury: a prospective study with comparison group and one-year follow-up. Spine 1985;10:765.

14. Feurstein M, Beattie P. Biobehavioral factors affecting pain and disability in low back pain: mechanics and assessment. Phys Ther 1995;75:267.

15. Polatin PB, Kinney RK, Gatchel RJ. Psychiatric illness and chronic low-back pain: the mind and the spine—which goes first? Spine 1993;18:66.

16. Meilman PW. Chronic Pain: Treatment Considerations. In BP D'Orazio (ed), Back Pain Rehabilitation. Boston: Andover Medical Publishers, 1993;115.

17. Margolis S, Rabins PV. The Johns Hopkins White Papers: Depression and Anxiety. Baltimore: The John Hopkins Medical Institutions, 1997;8.

18. Matheson LN. Symptom Magnification Syndrome Casebook. Employment and Rehabilitation Institute of California, 1991. [Materials presented at workshop May 30, 1992, in Pittsburgh.]

19. King RB. Managing Symptom Magnification. In BP D'Orazio (ed), Back Pain Rehabilitation. Boston: Andover Medical Publishers, 1993;130.

20. Waddell G, McCulloch JA, Kummel E, et al. Nonorganic physical signs in low back pain. Spine 1979;5:111.

21. Bigos SJ, Battie MC, Spengler DM, et al. A prospective study of work perceptions and psychosocial factors affecting the report of back injury. Spine 1991;16:1.

22. Klenerman L, Slade PD, Stanley IM, et al. The prediction of chronicity in patients with an acute attack of low back pain in a general practice setting. Spine 1995;20:478.

23. Hazard RG, Bendix A, Fenwick JW. Disability exaggeration as a predictor of functional restoration outcomes for patients with chronic low-back pain. Spine 1991;16:1062.

6

Exercise Prescription for Nonsurgical Low Back Pain Patients

Brian P. D'Orazio

Effects of Exercise on Acute and Chronic Low Back Pain

Exercise is widely prescribed and well validated for the treatment of low back pain (LBP). Haldeman stated that "[t]here is now a convincing body of research that demonstrates that strengthening exercise together with improvement of cardiovascular fitness and general functional restoration can reduce disability and possibly pain in patients with chronic low back pain."[1] As discussed in Chapter 5, the most successful strategies for treatment of chronic LBP patients include a combination of psychosocial support, quantitative testing, and exercise prescribed and supervised by a physical therapist.[2–13] A minimum of 2–3 months of rehabilitation is required to have lasting effects on patients with chronic LBP.[9,14,15] *Furthermore, patients must be allowed to continue in a rehabilitation program as long as there is objective evidence of continuing functional gains.*[15]

The efficacy of exercise programs on patients with acute and subacute LBP, until recently, has been disputed because of a lack of scientific evidence. Research published since 1990 on the effects of exercise for this patient population has established that properly prescribed exercise is efficacious both in reducing pain and in returning patients to work faster than traditional medical approaches.[6,16–18]

Although there currently is little dispute that exercise is extremely beneficial in the treatment of patients with LBP regardless of symptom duration, the specific prescription of exercise remains less clear. For both surgically treated and nonsurgically treated patients, adequate intensity is necessary.[7,14,16,19] Limiting exercise based only on the patients' report of pain is unwarranted.[20,21]

Strength and its relationship to LBP are well established among patients with chronic LBP. Multiple studies have demonstrated decreased muscle mass, diminished force production, diminished lower extremity strength, and diminished cardiovascular endurance.[3,7,22–24] The relationship of strength and LBP among patients with acute and subacute symptoms is not as clear. Evidence indicates that exercise programs are effective in preventing workers from losing time at work because of LBP and insufficient strength for a given task increases the incidence of LBP among workers.[18,25–27] But these studies do not answer the question of whether pre-existing strength deficits or other specific problems may predispose individuals to LBP.

Evaluation of Movement and Its Utility in Exercise Prescription

"Movement, whether purposeful or nonpurposeful, gross or fine, passive or active, is the common denominator to all therapeutic exercise interventions. Physical evaluations assess movements, then correlate movements with reports of pain in an attempt to diagnose the problem. Assumptions about the evaluation, such as the patient demonstrates his full capabilities, pain accurately reflects the patient's pathology, muscles always function synchronously to control movement, etc., are not always correct. For example, the problem created by symptom magnification is readily appreciated when attempting to prescribe treatment, as pain is often an inaccurate reflection of pathology. Equally inaccurate is the view that all abnormal movement patterns are the result of joint mechanical dysfunction. For this view to be valid, the given imperative would be that an individual's choice of movement pattern is predetermined by spinal mechanics."[28]

Furthermore, "[b]oth the lack of diagnostic value in the patient's pain report and our current inability to relate movement and pathology create a dilemma in clinical examination. On the one hand, presumptions that are scientifically invalidated may lead to erroneous conclusions; on the other hand, relying on what is known may render us incapable of performing a clinically useful examination. If, however, the issue of pathology is discarded for the moment, it may be possible to determine how movement is involved in the patient's pain complaint. The value of this determination, given that most of the time a definitive diagnosis is not possible, lies in the prescription of treatment."[28]

The remainder of this chapter considers two possible movement types referred to as *static dysfunctions* and *dynamic dysfunctions*. Typically, one of these movement types predominates. Nevertheless, the treatment of dynamic dysfunctions must precede the treatment of static dysfunctions if effective treatment is to be rendered. These classifications make no attempt to diagnose the underlying pathologic condition; rather, these movement types assist in the prescription of exercise.

Static Dysfunctions

Patients with static dysfunctions have as their predominant clinical picture the presence of iatrogenic changes in tissues that have created one or more problems relevant to their chief complaint, including weakness predominantly caused by muscle atrophy, soft-tissue restrictions, or instabilities. Patients with predominantly static dysfunctions are usually able to move near the end of their available range before experiencing significant pain. "[T]heir movement pattern, even if slightly guarded, is fairly well coordinated. These patients may forward bend only to the midtibial region; however, they are able to achieve that range before encountering great difficulty and they are then able to reassume an erect posture with minimal substitutive patterns. On further examination, the reason for the restricted motion is often clear; that is, some structures such as the hamstrings or back extensors are inflexible independent from the pain response."[28]

Dynamic Dysfunctions

Patients with predominantly dynamic dysfunctions are characterized by the demonstration of poorly coordinated movements that usually are very restricted with pain throughout most of the motion. A typical example is the patient who forward bends to about the knees and then is unable to continue with further movement, complains that pain exists throughout the entire range available, and has to push up off the legs in order to reassume an erect posture. Although the patient's active motion is extremely restricted, passively, the patient possesses component movements that would predict much greater ranges. Often, these patients present with 80 degrees of straight leg raising, 120 degrees of hip flexion, and adequate intersegmental lumbar motion to allow for full forward bending. Even in patients with extremely restricted motion segment mechanics, the presence of adequate hamstring and hip extensor length should allow the patient to forward bend well beyond the knees.

Patients with dynamic movement dysfunctions often report that pain limits their movement. In my experience, the dynamic dysfunction itself is actually a component of the patient's pain, perpetuating the symptoms. With adequate prescription, most of these patients will achieve nearly full range of motion within less than an hour without manual techniques. Typically after achieving this range, the patient reports a substantial reduction in pain, which supports the concept that the dynamic dysfunction perpetuates the pain complaint. "It is important to recognize pain as a symptom of dysfunction, not necessarily reflecting the severity of the pathology. For example, a cramp in the ankle plantar flexors is most certainly a painful phenomenon, but it is rare that the cramp itself is serious."[28]

Combined Dysfunctions

As stated previously, although static and dynamic movement dysfunctions are often concurrent, the dynamic dysfunction must resolve before the static dysfunction is treated. If an attempt is made to have the patient stretch the erector spinae while he or she possesses a substantial dynamic movement dysfunction, the patient will typically experience an increase in symptoms. Fortunately, dynamic dysfunctions usually can be resolved quickly, typically within one to five visits.

"Viewing dysfunction in this manner does not alter any eventual hypothesis regarding a diagnosis, nor does it infringe on any specific philosophies such as osteopathic, McKenzie, Paris, or others. Rather, it organizes the clinical approach, allowing the clinician to make reasonable judgments about the type of therapeutic exercise intervention to be used and how treatment should be sequenced."[28] By combining movement examination with other components of the physical examination and establishing a preliminary hypothesis regarding the underlying problem (mechanical dysfunctions, disc lesions, muscle spasms, inflammation, etc.) decisions about other therapeutic interventions are facilitated. Examples of static and dynamic exercises are contained in Appendix 6-1, at the end of this chapter.

Dynamic Exercise Prescription

Patient education, as in all phases of LBP treatment, is the key to success in prescription of a dynamic exercise regimen. Although pathologic involvement is not necessarily accurately portrayed by the extent of a patient's pain complaint, his or her anxiety usually is. For those patients with a substantial dynamic movement dysfunction, not only is pain usually affecting all aspects of their life, but they are also severely disabled by this condition. Patients with substantial dynamic movement dysfunctions typically have very high Oswestry scores.

Analogies of common conditions are often helpful in assisting the patient with becoming compliant with your request to engage in an exercise program. For patients with LBP and a dynamic movement dysfunction, an analogy between the severe pain associated with a calf cramp and the patient's LBP helps the patient understand why he or she must move in order to resolve the symptoms. Because the number of joints involved are few and the muscle is fairly simple, most people will instinctively be able to get rid of a cramp in their calf. The back, however, is a more complex structure, so there is little innate sense of how to relieve spasms, and hence these conditions are perpetuated. Patients are then told that the exercises which are prescribed for this condition help alleviate spasm and subsequently their discomfort. It is essential that the patient understand that the pain cannot be eliminated before movement patterns are normalized.

The patient must be offered a plausible explanation for the symptoms before he or she engages in a rigorous program to regain control of function. The clinician's hypothesis regarding the actual reason for the patient's problem is not as important as making that explanation relevant to the exercises being prescribed and working with the patient's perception of his or her pathologic condition. Even within the context of a disc lesion, movement dysfunctions can occur and the patient needs to understand that he or she can safely overcome the movement component of the problem without producing a negative impact on his or her injured disc.

The specific prescription of exercise is dependent on the restriction of movements. Patients with dynamic movement dysfunctions typically are tender to palpation in a large area. Most of the time, there is considerable co-contraction of the flexors and extensors of the trunk. If there is too much involvement in the hip flexor musculature, sometimes asking the patient to repetitively flex will exacerbate his or her symptoms. Under these circumstances, extension should be the first exercise prescribed. Flexion usually is the first direction prescribed and needs to be achieved successfully before pushing substantially into extension.

Based on the clinician's evaluation and after the patient has been offered an explanation of why this particular series of exercises is being prescribed, the first movement typically is repetitive quadruped flexion (Figure 6A-1). Usually, the movement is repeated 15 times, encouraging the patient to move either in pain-free ranges or with minimal discomfort. Manual contacts may be necessary to guide movement (Figure 6A-2). Assistance should not be perceived as forcing movement but rather as providing manual cues to help the patient understand how to move.

Repetitive seated flexion is the next movement performed (Figure 6A-3). Initially the patient may need to push off the knees in order to accomplish this movement. Once the patient has become more proficient in this movement, the patient should be encouraged to slide the hands between the legs, gradually reaching the floor (Figure 6A-4). Some patients may actually perform this activity more easily than quadruped flexion; for others the reverse will be true. Again, the movement is usually performed for 15 repetitions per set.

For most patients, it is important that both quadruped and seated flexion are achieved successfully through nearly full ranges before progressing to the next series of movements. For some patients this is as far as one can go with the first day of rehabilitation. Often, four or five sets of each movement with verbal and even manual assistance are required to achieve full range movement. If after several sets the patient is still not moving through nearly normal ranges, it may be necessary to encourage the patient to engage the pain with movement.

The next phase of movement is standing lateral flexion (Figure 6A-5). If the patient has difficulty maintaining movement in a frontal plane, having the patient initially stand against the wall will help pattern the motion. Usually by the time lateral flexion is started, some success has already been achieved with the previous two movements. Additionally, lateral flexion is not as difficult to control as flexion. For both reasons, the patient usually is not as anxious at this time.

Initially, the patient is not allowed to forward bend beyond the knees and the patient's movement is gradually sequenced until he or she is able to touch the floor and reassume an erect posture without pushing off the legs and with good control (Figure 6A-6). The movement is repeated 10–15 times per set based on physical findings and the patient's performance. If the patient moves into a range that he or she cannot control, the patient will experience pain and then cannot reassume an erect posture without assisting himself or herself by pushing off the legs. The clinician needs to further restrict the patient's movements while encouraging the patient to gradually go further once he or she has achieved better control.

After each standing flexion, standing backward bending is performed (Figure 6A-7). These movements must be controlled, must be initially pain free, and must be sequenced to gradually increase movement. Usually by this stage in the rehabilitation program, the patient has been successful enough with movements that he or she is more willing to engage some discomfort, realizing that the ability to increase range of motion is of assistance in reducing the symptoms.

Once the patient is able to move through a full range of motion in quadruped and seated flexion and is able to forward bend to the ankles and backward bend 5 degrees or more while standing, prone press-ups are added (Figure 6A-8). Once the patient is able to perform full-range prone extensions, quadruped flexion/extension is prescribed (Figure 6A-9). Manual contacts are often needed initially to achieve a controlled movement sequence (Figure 6A-10).

Once the patient has achieved full range of motion in each position and can perform 15 repetitions with good form, he or she is progressed to light weights. The entire sequence is sometimes achieved within the first treatment session. For most patients, however, this is not prescribed until the second or third visit.

The addition of light weights adds to the complexity of the task and therefore requires a higher level of neuromuscular organization than was previously required. Figure 6A-11 depicts the initial movement of standing forward bending using a 5-pound dumbbell held vertically. The dumbbell will limit range of motion, allowing the patient to become comfortable with the new task. The knees remain flexed during this motion, and lumbar flexion is encouraged. This helps improve control of lumbar flexion. In most cases, flexion of the lumbar spine is safe with very light loads as long as the motion is well controlled. When heavier weights are used, however, this would not be the position of choice for the lumbar spine, as will be discussed later in this chapter.

Once the patient is able to move pain free and touch the end of the dumbbell to the floor for 15 repetitions, the patient progresses to holding the dumbbell parallel to the floor (Figure 6A-12). Before progressing beyond this stage of rehabilitation, the patient must be able to perform 20 repetitions, with the 5-pound weight held horizontally for two sets, without pain either during movement or pain the following day associated with this exercise. It is extremely important that this movement is fluid and painless before the patient progresses. This may require several additional sessions.

The next movement is standing lateral trunk bends using 5 pounds of resistance (Figure 6A-13). This movement is usually well tolerated, but the patient should not progress to it until a minimum of two consecutive sets of 20 repetitions through a full range of motion are performed without pain. The patient should not experience pain the following day, and the decision to progress the patient to the next weight therefore is held until that time.

The next movement prescribed is active lumbar extension (hyperextensions) against gravity (Figure 6A-14). If the patient has considerable spasm in the lumbar erector spinae, this movement initially should not be prescribed. Once the patient has been successful with the other exercises, however, active lumbar extension will further help in reducing lumbar erector spinae pain.

The Home Program

Table 6-1 illustrates the typical prescription of a home program for patients with dynamic movement dysfunctions. This table describes all the exercises performed without weights, but the prescription should be for only those movements that are appropriate. Often, only quadruped and seated flexion are initially prescribed. The exercises are prescribed for every 30 minutes, over the next 6 hours after the first visit, if the movement dysfunction

Table 6-1 Home Prescription: Dynamic Movement Program

Movement	Repetitions	Frequency and sets
Quadruped flexion	15–20	1–2 sets every 30 mins for 6 hrs and then 1–2 sets every hour thereafter until otherwise prescribed
Seated flexion	15–20	1–2 sets every 30 mins for 6 hrs and then 1–2 sets every hour thereafter until otherwise prescribed
Standing lateral flexion	15–20	1–2 sets every 30 mins for 6 hrs and then 1–2 sets every hour thereafter until otherwise prescribed
Standing flexion and extension	10–15	1–2 sets every 30 mins for 6 hrs and then 1–2 sets every hour thereafter until otherwise prescribed
Prone press-ups	15–20	1–2 sets every 30 mins for 6 hrs and then 1–2 sets every hour thereafter until otherwise prescribed
Quadruped flexion and extension	10–15	1–2 sets every 30 mins for 6 hrs and then 1–2 sets every hour thereafter until otherwise prescribed

is severe. If the movement dysfunction is not as severe, the patient performs the exercises at least hourly for sets of 15–20 repetitions. If only quadruped and seated flexion are performed initially, two sets of each exercise should be performed at each session. The first home session must begin as soon as the patient walks through the door of his or her home. I admonish patients not to take side trips or run errands on the first day. Usually, even a 5-minute ride in the car will make the patient feel "stiff." For this reason, going to the grocery store or making a trip to the mall will exacerbate the condition, making performance of the prescribed exercises more difficult. Under most circumstances, it is ideal to see the patient for his or her second visit the next day. Patients are usually compliant with the request to perform exercises every 30 minutes because, if appropriately prescribed, this movement significantly reduces the pain, and between sessions patients feel themselves losing motion and having more pain.

Once the patient begins to move more normally, it is not uncommon that some benign movement during an activity of daily living will cause a sharp pain. I find this to be true in approximately 20% of my patients. As a consequence, I warn every patient that if he or she experiences a sharp pain, the patient should immediately get in the quadruped flexion position and repetitively perform quadruped flexions until he or she feels that control of movement has been achieved, and then the patient should sequence through the program the same way that it was originally prescribed. I further tell the patient that the sharp pain is likely muscular, it probably represents some type of a spasm, and just as the patient was told with cramps, it should be eliminated as soon as possible to avoid further pain.

Management Considerations for Patients with Dynamic Movement Dysfunctions

Patients who do not achieve nearly normal control of these initial movements within four visits often have a substantial psychosocial component to their pathologic state. If the clinician is still convinced that a more serious pathologic condition does not exist, referral of that patient to a mental health professional is essential. Continuing these patients in treatment without such a referral will be frustrating for the clinician and the patient.

There are many techniques that can be used to achieve normal trunk neuromuscular control. The approach that I use is basic and easy to teach, and the progression is rapid. These movement techniques establish basic gross motor skills. Once gross motor skills are achieved, the clinician can begin working on fine trunk motor skills, such as cats and camels, alternate arm and leg raises from a quadruped position, or a variety of exercises sometimes performed on a therapeutic ball. It is not necessarily essential to prescribe each of these fine motor coordination skills, but depending on the patient's condition and the preference of the therapist, any of these activities or others can be prescribed at this time. Additionally, the patient can usually begin a stretching program, but I start with simple stretches such as hamstring or hip external rotator stretching and make sure that these are successful before progressing to stretching of the erector spinae.

Prescription of Exercise for Static Dysfunctions

Static exercise prescription begins after the patient has achieved mastery of gross motor skills. At this time, the remaining deficits should be primarily related to the static conditions previously described. If the problem was dynamic and the patient's condition is relatively acute, there may not be a need for static exercise prescription. If the dynamic dysfunction was small or nonexistent, the prescription of exercises should immediately address the static components that are contributing to the patient's chief complaint.

Flexibility

If the patient had a substantial dynamic component to the movement dysfunction, the clinician may not have been able to fully examine flexibility, which should now be evaluated. Initially, prescribing stretching exercises should be limited to only those muscle groups that the clinician thinks most directly relate to the patient's chief complaint. The fact that a muscle is inflexible does not necessarily mean that stretching for that muscle group needs to be performed immediately; however, inflexibility of certain muscle groups, such as the hip external rotators, hip flexors, the lumbar erector spinae, or the hamstrings, are typically of primary concern. Initially, the clinician must limit the number of stretches prescribed. This helps control variables, which promotes better decision making. Typically, no more than three or four stretches are initially prescribed. There are many reasons for this, but one of the reasons is that patients often stretch too aggressively and exacerbate symptoms. Limiting the number of stretches helps the clinician control this problem.

The amount of specific research into the use of stretching to treat LBP is limited. Although stretching is a commonly performed technique, Khalil and colleagues are some of the few authors to formally study the effects of stretching on LBP.[29] The specific techniques used by the authors, however, were manual and progressive, demonstrating excellent efficacy. In the following sections, the primary emphasis is on the prescription of stretching as a self-management exercise.

Back Extensors

Because of multiple fiber directions in the back extensors, a multitude of stretches can be used. It is important that the clinician evaluate which portion of the back extensors is most in need of stretching and that the stretches change according to the patient's progression. Although all stretches initially must be comfortable, patients must gradually progress through greater ranges to achieve a more desirable flexibility. Figure 6A-15 demonstrates common positions for stretching the back extensors. Only the most appropriate positions should be chosen based on a wide range of clinical variables. Manual stretches are sometimes required to achieve increased flexibility in specific areas but will not be discussed in this chapter.

Trunk Flexors

The iliopsoas is commonly involved in back dysfunction. Figure 6A-16 depicts a common position for stretching the iliopsoas, although the emphasis in this position is clearly on the iliacus. Figure 6A-17 adds a rotational component to the stretch that seems to more effectively stretch the psoas major along with the iliacus. Figure 6A-18 is another general hip flexor stretch that more specifically targets the proximal rectus femoris but with some skill can be made to stretch both the iliacus and the psoas major.

Abdominal contractures are rare but can be found in some runners and in abdominal surgery patients. Figure 6A-19 demonstrates a stretch for the rectus abdominis.

Hip Abductors, Hip External Rotators, Hip Extensors, Hamstrings, and Ankle Plantar Flexors

The stretches for the hip abductors, hip external rotators, hip extensors, hamstrings, and ankle plantar flexors are generally well understood by clinicians, and therefore the primary instructions for these exercises in this chapter are included in Figures 6A-20 to 6A-31. Of these, the hip abductors are probably the most difficult stretches to perform. Additionally, the hip abductor stretches should not be prescribed when patients have substantial amounts of lumbar pain, because stretch positions for the hip abductors typically stress the lumbar spine in both the frontal and horizontal planes.

General Management Strategies for Stretching

Most articles on stretching emphasize static versus ballistic stretching as being relatively safer and more effective. Patients should be instructed to relax while stretching, to hold a stretch position for 40 seconds, to release from the stretched position for at least 10 seconds before performing another repetition, and to repeat the stretch three times. The frequency per day should be varied according to the results desired. Usually I have patients stretch three times a day initially, and within the first week I decrease this to twice a day and then maintain the patient at once a day. Variations on this prescription are based, as expected, on the patient's condition.

Strength Training

Strength training, as with stretching, depends on sound clinical judgment augmented by personal experience. There is a substantial research base that has examined trunk strength as a variable in low back pain.[30–33] Which specific exercises to prescribe, how much weight to prescribe, how far the patient should be progressed, and many other issues have yet to be specifically defined by research. Knowledge about exercise training for the trunk, the lower extremities, and the upper extremities, however, is substantial because of sports programs and adaptations of sports-specific programs to therapeutic interventions by physical therapists and other professionals.

"Training programs for patients differ from training programs for athletes primarily in intensity. All programs must be tailored to the severity of involvement and to the patient's previous experience with exercise. Relatively high repetitions should be used per set when working with patients. This decreases the intensity of the contraction and consequently lowers the risk of re-injury. In the early phases of weight training for patients, the benefit comes not so much from challenging the muscles but rather in training the body to move."[28]

Patients who are either anxious about exercise or extremely deconditioned benefit by starting with only one set of relatively few exercises. This should minimize normal exercise soreness, which some patients mistake for an exacerbation of their condition. For those patients who are fearful that the pain represents an extension of the pathologic condition, the exercise program needs to be progressed more slowly. It is important, however, to continue to progress these patients at every session. Even if the patient complains of more pain, it is important to reassure the patient that it is normal to experience minor pain with exercise. Even if the patient performs only one additional repetition per set of each exercise, the sense of accomplishment from having achieved the additional repetition and the probability that, in fact, the pain will have decreased after the next exercise session, will reinforce the need for the patient to exercise.

For most patients, two sets of exercise can initially be prescribed. The patient should be told to anticipate some minor exercise-related soreness and most people will understand that concept. When treating chronic pain patients, refer to Chapter 5 for advice on how to manage those patients' conditions. Once the patient no longer experiences exercise soreness from two sets and after the weights have been increased successfully for several sessions, it may be necessary to progress the patient to three sets per exercise, depending on the patient's condition and functional needs.

Clinicians must keep in mind the relative percentage increase of weights when making determinations of how much to increase the weight. For example, if the patient is lifting 100 pounds of weight for some specific exercise, an increase of 10 pounds is a small percentage increase, whereas a patient who moves from 20 pounds to 30 pounds in an exercise experiences a large percentage increase. If patients have problems transitioning to an increased weight, keeping the patient at a lower weight but increasing repetitions for a time usually helps to advance the weight.

For all patients, progress is documented by using exercise charts (Figure 6A-32). Room is left at the end of the chart to write in specific exercises that are less commonly prescribed. Each exercise session contains data about the weight used in a exercise, the repetitions per set of each exercise, and the date of the session. Notations can be made on the chart to help guide exercise prescription at the next session.

Hyperextensions

One of the most effective exercises for the lower lumbar erector spinae is hyperextensions. As previously described in this chapter, hyperextensions are started with the patient's hands behind his or her back (see Figure 6A-14). To progress the patient in this exercise, the patient must be able to move through his or her full range of motion for at least two sets of between 20 and 30 repetitions. I usually use 30 repetitions per set as the standard for hyperextensions throughout all progressions of this exercise. I believe that 30 repetitions per set stimulate both type I and type II fiber recruitment. Figure 6A-33 depicts a logical sequence of progression for hyperextensions. If necessary, weights can also be held to the chest once the patient has successfully completed sets of 30 repetitions on the Roman chair with the hands behind the neck. Clinicians must never assume that because the patient has successfully completed one exercise he or she will continue using good form throughout the next progression of the exercise. Consequently, observation and palpation are frequently necessary.

Abdominal Training

Common abdominal exercises are depicted in Figure 6A-34. There are many variations on these exercises, far too many to include in this text. The abdominals are part of a complex mechanical system of support for the lumbar spine. Contraction of the abdominals pulls on the thoracodorsal fascia, which is thought to support the lumbar spine. Although the precise mechanism is unclear, the importance of abdominal training is not disputed by many clinicians or researchers.

Usually, abdominal exercises are progressed by increasing repetitions. Again, form and technique are important. Patients can easily strain the cervical spine if it is weak, poorly supported, or if poor technique is used. Each of the exercises should be performed slowly, moving to the end of the range with good muscular control, not momentum.

Trunk Flexors

The role of the iliopsoas in stabilizing and moving the lumbar spine is generally well understood, although its location makes research difficult. Because of the relatively limited research on this muscle and its remote access to clinical examination, this muscle group is unfortunately not considered in many rehabilitation programs. The iliopsoas is responsible for much of the range of movement into lumbar flexion that occurs when a subject performs a full-range sit-up; however, because of the potential harm that can occur to the lumbar spine in performing full-range sit-ups, this activity has almost been abandoned.[34] With proper supervision and instruction, this exercise can be performed safely and effectively (Figure 6A-35). This activity is not necessary for most patients but is included in this chapter for the sake of completeness. Generally, activities such as straight leg raises, stationary cycling, and other activities are probably adequate for training this group of muscles.

Lateral Trunk Bends

Lateral trunk bends were described previously and depicted in Figure 6A-13. Clinicians must be vigilant in supervising this activity so the patients continue moving in a frontal plane. Additionally, patients often lose range of motion as they increase weight, and again the clinician is instrumental in guiding the patient through an adequate amount of range that is consistent from session to session.

Dead Lifts

As noted previously, "[d]ead lifts are probably the most controversial exercise in the rehabilitation of LBP patients. If properly performed, the motion is safe and is the primary exercise to help prepare for normal lifting activities."[28] Because of the fear of injuring a disc when performing this activity, the common prohibitions against this type of lifting often limit the patient's ability to progress in rehabilitation. When performed properly, this is an extremely safe technique, as evidenced by many weight lifters who lift hundreds of pounds. If patients are untrained in this exercise, however, they almost certainly will injure their back when they return to this type of activity. When performed with proper form, a complex movement that integrates lower extremity function with trunk motion will be patterned through dead lifts. This should carry over to routine lifting during activities of daily living and is an excellent exercise for strengthening the lower thoracic and upper lumbar erector spinae.

Dead lifts are best progressed by having the patient hold a dumbbell vertically as mentioned earlier in this chapter. As soon as the patient progresses to use of a 10-pound dumbbell, the form for this activity changes from the form used during the dynamic movement exercises (see Figure 6A-11). I typically progress the patient to a 45-pound olympic bar after the patient has been successful in repetitively lifting a 30-pound dumbbell, even though this is a substantial increase in weight. Probably because of the difference in weight distribution, most patients are not even aware that they are lifting a heavier weight when they go to the olympic bar. Sound clinical judgment needs to be used before making this progression in weight.

As depicted in Figures 6A-36 and 6A-37, there are two primary methods for performing dead lifts using an olympic bar. The conventional style of dead lift is common in competition but does not have as much practical application for patient training, whereas the sumo style emphasizes hip abduction, which is a more typical position to use when performing routine lifting or manual materials handling. Clinicians should have substantial experience in lifting techniques when instructing patients in this difficult but extremely beneficial exercise.

Other Exercises

Upper and lower extremity exercises are also important in the overall reconditioning program for patients with LBP. This is especially true for patients with chronic LBP. For all patients, however, the latissimus dorsi are used both in protection of the low back and in initiation of certain rapid movements. Typical exercises for the latissimus dorsi are depicted in Figures 6A-38 and 6A-39. Another reason for upper extremity strengthening is to decrease the load on the lumbar spine. I find that women particularly rely more heavily on the back and lower extremities during lifting because of relatively weak upper extremities. Furthermore, some LBP patients have other problems with their upper extremities that have caused them to emphasize lifting with their legs or back, which may predispose them to injuries.

Lower extremity strengthening is of more obvious benefit than upper extremity training. One of the most beneficial lower extremity exercises is the squat. I progress patients through this exercise sequentially, starting with limited range squats that are specifically measured and then progressing to squats that typically bring them to approximately 90 degrees of knee flexion. Figure 6A-40 demonstrates proper form for a dumbbell squat. I never recommend using a bar behind the neck for performaing squats by patients with LBP.

Another excellent exercise that combines lower extremity training with trunk stabilization is the lunge. Figure 6A-41 depicts this exercise performed with a weight, but typically the exercise is initially performed without the weight.

Other exercises commonly used include leg curls, leg extensions, standing calf raises, and functionally specific exercises along with many others depending on the needs of the patient. The time involved in exercise must be considered. I minimize relatively peripheral routines that do not have a direct impact on the patient's chief complaints.

Endurance Training

It is important to consider both cardiovascular and muscular endurance in a patient's rehabilitation program. Back extensor endurance training is particularly important and often overlooked. High repetitions of exercises such as hyperextensions on the Roman chair, repetitive lifting, and training in sustained forward-bent postures are excellent activities for increasing endurance of the lumbar erector spinae. Considering that type I muscle fiber atrophy is common in patients with LBP, retraining the lumbar extensors to increase endurance may be one of the most critical factors in rehabilitation. Additionally, activities such as walking also help to increase not only the patient's endurance for walking but also endurance for sitting. The ability to lift weight should not be confused with the patient's ability to perform some other activity. I have had many patients who could lift 150 pounds, yet they were unable to tolerate a forward-flexed position for more than 30 seconds. A sustained horizontal position off the Roman chair is an excellent means for increasing back endurance, and this is one of the more heavily researched positions for that purpose. I typically try to increase endurance time to at least 2 minutes and incorporate this as a separate exercise at the end of two or three sets of hyperextensions.

Cardiovascular endurance training is well understood by all physical therapists. There are many pieces of equipment for this purpose, but exercise bicycles, treadmills, and stair-stepping machines are most commonly used. Patients should not simply use these pieces of equipment to occupy time. Specific goals need to be set, and the patient needs to be exercised in target zones for prescribed time frames. Heart rate monitoring equipment can help in this process if necessary. I usually have patients exercise on multiple pieces of equipment for up to 20 minutes for the cross-training effect. The exception is walking, which I prefer to have patients do outside, and they are progressed up to 4 miles per walk.

Conclusion

"[E]xercise prescriptions need to move toward simplicity. Exercises should be easily understood by clinicians and most importantly, by patients."[28] As in many phases of rehabilitation, personal experience with all exercises is important. If you have not experienced the exercise, you cannot adequately instruct the patient in that exercise. Furthermore, clinicians should be actively involved in their patients' exercise programs. Although support personnel may be used in supervising exercise programs, the clinician should observe movements and palpate during exercise to ensure that appropriate muscle groups are used and that patients are safe in all phases of that program. With a full knowledge of patients' pathologic conditions, their ability to move, and their psychosocial condition, proper prescription of exercise for patients with LBP is perhaps the most powerful clinical tool that a physical therapist can possess.

References

1. Haldeman S. Presidential Address, North American Spine Society. Failure of the pathology model to predict back pain. Spine 1990;15:718.
2. Fordyce WE, McMahon R, Rainwater G, et al. Pain complaint: exercise performance relationship in chronic pain. Pain 1981;10:311.
3. Mayer TG, Gatchel RJ, Kishino N, et al. Objective assessment of spine function following industrial injury: a prospective study with comparison group and one-year follow-up. Spine 1985;10:482.
4. Alston W, Carlson KE, Feldman D, et al. A quantitative study of muscle factors in the chronic low-back syndrome. J Am Geriatr Soc 1966;14:1041.
5. Nicolaisen T, Jorgensen T. Trunk strength, back muscle endurance and low-back trouble. Scand J Rehab Med 1985;14:121.
6. Lindstrom I, Ohlund C, Eek C, et al. The effect of graded activity on patients with subacute low back pain: a randomized prospective clinical study with an operant conditioning behavioral approach. Phys Ther 1992;72:279.
7. Rissanen A, Kalimo H, Alaranta H. Effect of intensive training on the isokinetic strength and structure of lumbar muscles in patients with chronic low back pain. Spine 1995;20:333.
8. Lanes TC, Gauron EF, Spratt KF, et al. Long-term follow-up of patients with chronic back pain treated in a multidisciplinary rehabilitation program. Spine 1995;20:801.
9. Reilly K, Lovejoy B, Williams R, Roth H. Differences between a supervised and independent strength and conditioning program with chronic low back syndromes. J Occup Med 1989;31:547.
10. Rainville J, Ahern DK, Phalen L, et al. The association of pain with physical activities in chronic low back pain. Spine 1992;17:1060.
11. Garcy P, Mayer TG, Gatchel RJ. Recurrent or new injury outcomes after return to work in chronic disabling spinal disorders: tertiary prevention efficacy of functional restoration treatment. Spine 1996;21:952.
12. Hazard RG, Bendix A, Fenwick JW. Disability exaggeration as a predictor of functional restoration outcomes for patients with chronic low back pain. Spine 1991;19:1062.

13. Mayer TG, Polatin P, Smith B, et al. Contemporary concepts in spine care, spine rehabilitation: secondary and tertiary nonoperative care. Spine 1995;20:2060.
14. Kellett KM, Kellett DA, Nordholm LA. Effects of an exercise program on sick leave due to back pain. Phys Ther 1991;71:283.
15. Hazard RG, Fenwick JW, Kalisch SM, et al. Functional restoration with behavioral support: a one-year prospective study of patients with chronic low-back pain. Spine 1989;14:157.
16. Mitchell RI, Carmen GM. Results of a multi-centered trial using an intensive active exercise program for the treatment of acute soft tissue and back injuries. Spine 1990;15:514.
17. Gundewall B, Liljeqvist M, Hansson T. Primary prevention of back symptoms and absence from work: a prospective randomized study among hospital employees. Spine 1993;18:587.
18. Ryan WE, Krishna MK, Swanson CE. A prospective study evaluating early rehabilitation in preventing back pain chronicity in mine workers. Spine 1995;20:489.
19. Manniche C, Asmussen K, Lauritsen B, et al. Intensive dynamic back exercises with or without hyperextension in chronic back pain after surgery for lumbar disc protrusion. Spine 1993;18:560.
20. Linton SJ. The relationship between activity and chronic back pain. Pain 1985;21:289.
21. Timm KE. Case Report: Use of Trunk Dynamometers in the Management of Patients with Spinal Disorders. In BP D'Orazio (ed), Back Pain Rehabilitation. Boston: Andover Medical Publishers, 1993;238.
22. Cady L, Bischoff D, O'Connel E, et al. Strength and fitness and subsequent back injuries in firefighters. J Occup Med 1979;21:269.
23. Flicker PL, Fleckenstein JL, Ferry K, et al. Lumbar muscle usage in chronic low back pain: magnetic resonance image evaluation. Spine 1993;18:582.
24. Leino P, Aro S, Hasan J. Trunk muscle function and low-back disorders: a 10-year follow-up study. J Chron Dis 1987;40:289.
25. Chaffin DB. Human strength capability and low back pain. J Occup Med 1974;16:248.
26. Keyserling WM, Herrin GD, Chaffin DB. Isometric strength testing as a means of controlling medical incidents on strenuous jobs. J Occup Med 1980;22:332.
27. Troup JDG, Martin JW, Lloyd DC. Back pain in industry. A prospective survey. Spine 1981;6:61.

28. D'Orazio BP. Exercise Prescription for Low Back Pain. In BP D'Orazio (ed), Back Pain Rehabilitation. Boston: Andover Medical Publishers, 1993;32.
29. Khalil TM, Asfour SS, Martinez LM, et al. Stretching in the rehabilitation of low-back pain patients. Spine 1992;17:311.
30. Flint MM. Effect of increasing back and abdominal muscle strength on low back pain. Res Quart 1955;24:160.
31. Langrana NA, Lee CK. Isokinetic evaluation of trunk muscles. Spine 1984;9:287.
32. Kishino ND, Mayer TG, Gatchel RJ, et al. Quantification of lumbar function. Part IV: isometric and isokinetic lifting simulation in normal subjects and low-back dysfunction patients. Spine 1985;10:921.
33. McNeill T, Warwick D, Andersson G, Ashultz A. Trunk strengths in attempted flexion, extension and lateral bending in healthy subjects and patients with low-back disorders. Spine 1980;5:529.
34. Andersson E, Oddsson L, Grundstrom H, Thorstensson A. The role of the psoas and iliacus muscles for stability and movement of the lumbar spine, pelvis and hip. Scand J Med Sci Sports 1995;5:10.

Chapter 6
Appendix

Appendix 6-1

Static and Dynamic Exercises

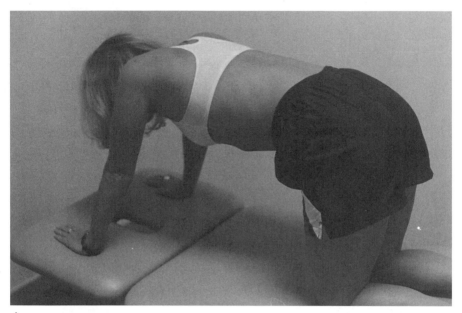

A

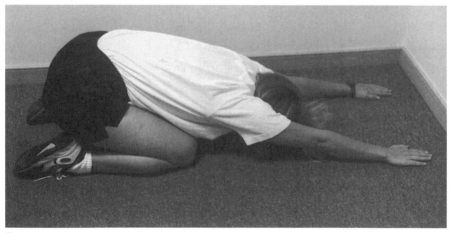

B

Figure 6A-1 (A) The patient begins in a quadruped position with the hands usually somewhat in front of the shoulders and the knees placed approximately at the same width as the shoulders. (B) When the patient has achieved full range of motion, the hand placement will naturally encourage flexion in the lumbar and thoracic spine. The cervical spine is fully flexed and the hips and knees are in full flexion at the end of the movement.

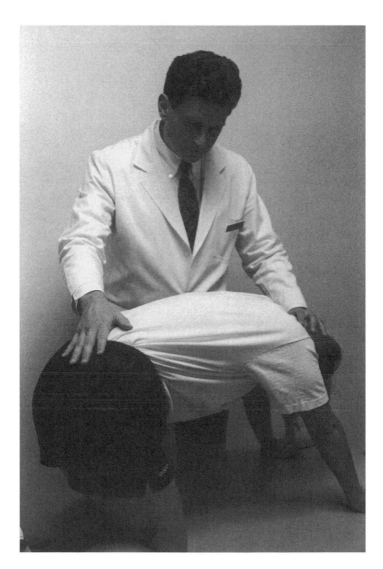

Figure 6A-2 Manual contacts may be necessary to guide movement. Hand placement is typically over the sacrum and on the patient's head. This reminds the patient to flex the cervical spine at the same time as he or she is flexing the hips.

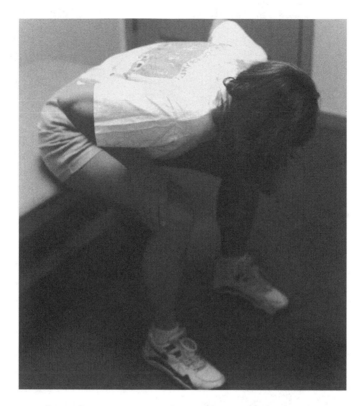

Figure 6A-3 Often, the patient must begin repetitive seated flexion by providing assistance with the arms. The clinician should verbally limit the patient's movements so he or she remains well controlled, gradually increasing the range until the patient can bring the chest to the knees and resume an erect posture when pushing off the knees without struggling.

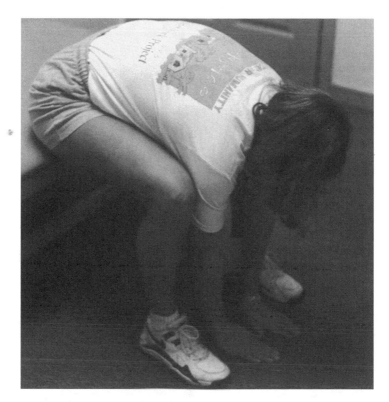

Figure 6A-4 Once the patient has successfully completed repetitive seated flexion with assistance, he or she is ready to begin gradually progressing into seated flexion without using the upper extremities for assistance. The clinician should assist the patient by allowing only controlled movements. Once several sets have been completed, if the patient is still reticent to move, the clinician may have to accept the patient initially losing some form to achieve greater range of motion.

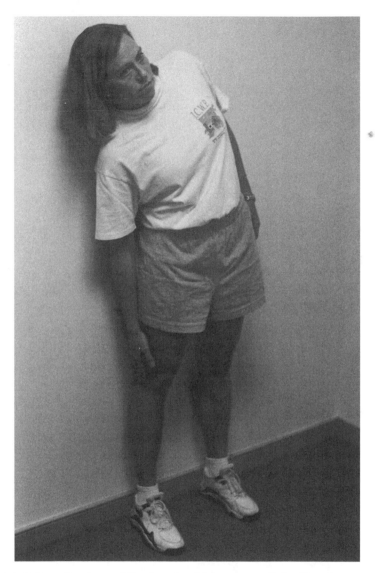

Figure 6A-5 Standing lateral flexion should be accomplished by slow controlled movements that remain in the frontal plane. Patients should maintain hand contacts along the iliotibial bands both to guide the movement and to help the clinician better visualize range of motion.

Figure 6A-6 (A) Standing flexion is accomplished by having the patient maintain contact with the anterior lower extremities, maintain a slightly flexed knee position throughout the range, flex the cervical spine, and initially restrict the movement so that the patient's hands only reach the knees. (B) Standing flexion is allowed to progress through a full range once the patient has sequentially demonstrated normal control of movement without exacerbating the pain. The patient's hands remain in contact with the lower extremities at all times.

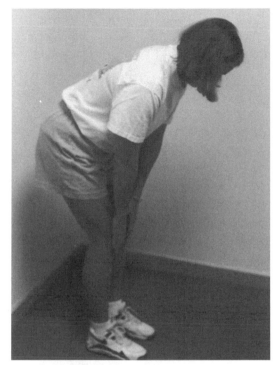

A

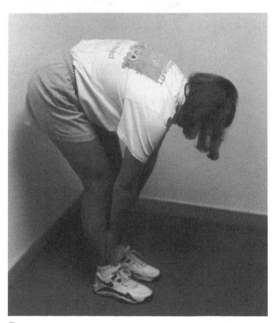

B

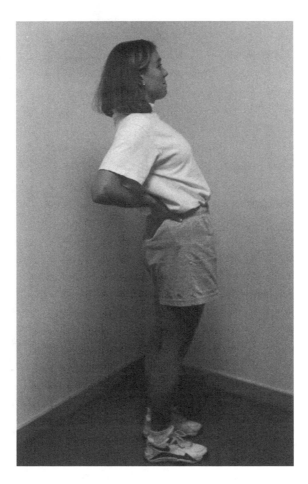

Figure 6A-7 Standing backward bending is performed after each forward-bending movement by having the patient place the hands as shown and requesting initially minimal movement. The transition from flexion to extension should be seamless, with the clinician giving continuous feedback about the quality and range of motion desired.

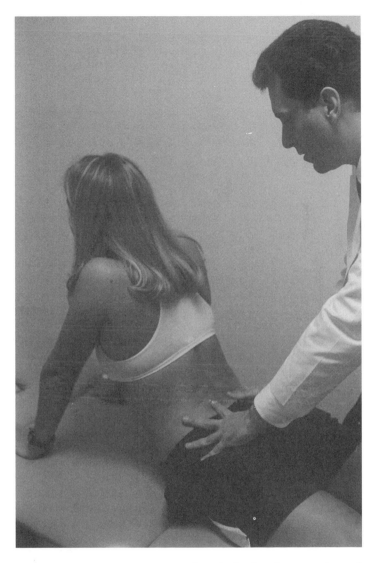

Figure 6A-8 Prone press-ups are initiated with the hands approximately parallel to the patient's eyes to assist in focusing motion on the lumbar spine. The therapist should palpate the pelvis and observe the lumbar spine to ensure that the desired movement is being achieved.

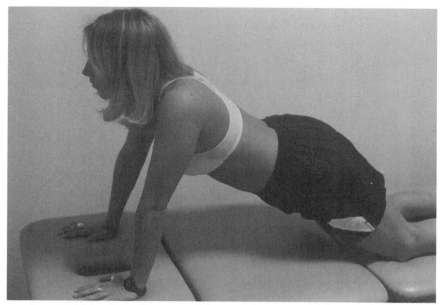

A

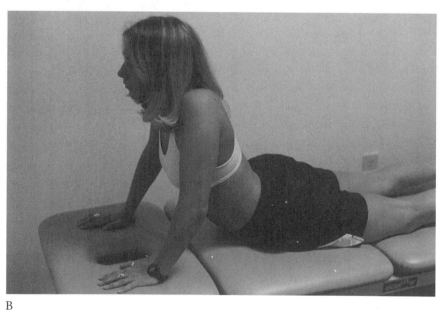

B

Figure 6A-9 (A) Quadruped extension begins with the hands slightly forward of the shoulders and the patient is encouraged to extend the cervical spine during the movement. (B) In full quadruped extension, the pelvis should be in contact with the ground, the elbows fully extended, and the cervical spine extended.

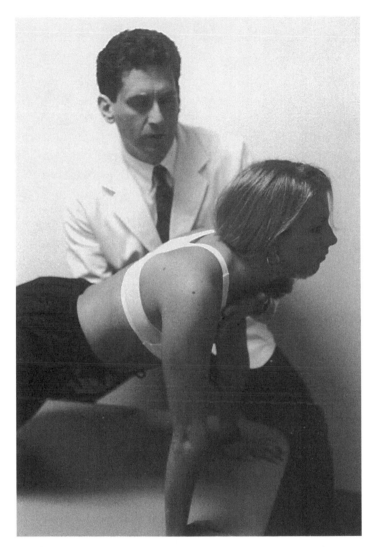

Figure 6A-10 The initial manual contacts for quadruped extension are on the patient's abdomen and chest. Commands are given to the patient to maintain elbow extension throughout the movement, to drop the pelvis, and to maintain cervical extension. In returning from quadruped extension, the contacts remain the same with enough support given by the clinician to assist the patient in smoothly transitioning back to a neutral quadruped position before moving into flexion.

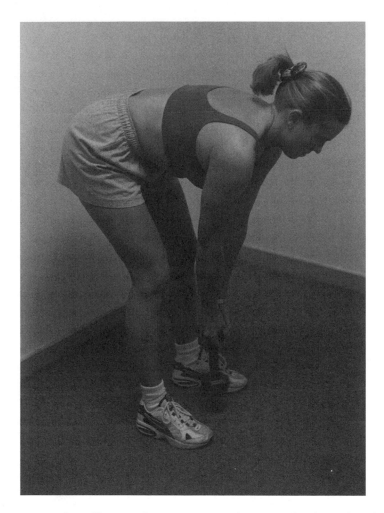

Figure 6A-11 Before allowing the patient to perform weighted standing forward bending, the therapist should demonstrate the motion, instructing the patient to keep the head of the dumbbell between the feet, maintain approximately 10 degrees of knee flexion, and move slowly through the range without pain.

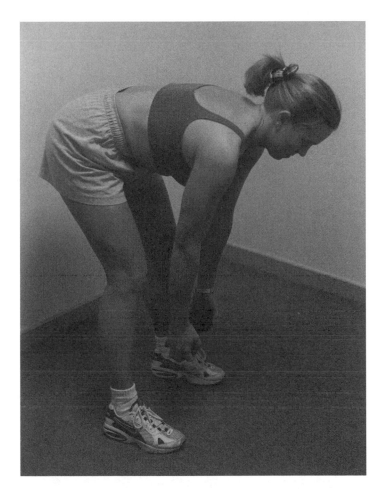

Figure 6A-12 Horizontal dumbbell lifts are performed according to the same variables as described when the dumbbell is held vertically. It is important that 10 degrees of knee flexion be maintained throughout the range and that the dumbbell is kept close to the body throughout the range. If the patient is unable to reassume an erect posture from a fully flexed position using the 5-pound weight, he or she is not ready to progress to holding the dumbbell horizontally and the clinician should return the patient to a vertical dumbbell position for several additional sets.

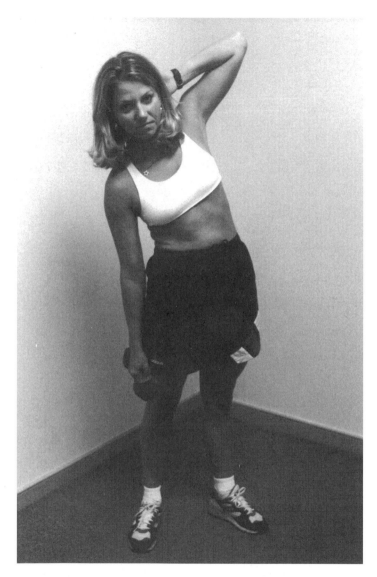

Figure 6A-13 Throughout lateral bending, the patient's hand should be in contact with the lateral thigh. The clinician should be vigilant about encouraging the patient to move only in the frontal plane and to move through as full a range as possible without pain. The resistance is not progressed until the patient is capable of accomplishing 20 repetitions for two sets through a full range without pain either the day of the exercise or the day after the exercise.

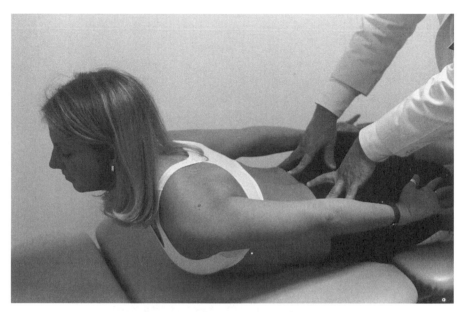

Figure 6A-14 Active lumbar extensions against gravity, referred to as *hyperextensions*, are performed on a surface that initially flexes the lumbar spine. The patient's hands are placed on the lumbar spine and the therapist gently palpates to ensure that the pelvis remains in contact with the surface and the movements are being accomplished only through the lumbar spine. Typically, two sets of 10 repetitions are prescribed initially, although fewer repetitions will be prescribed for some patients. No more than 10 repetitions are prescribed until the patient is capable of actively extending through the full available range.

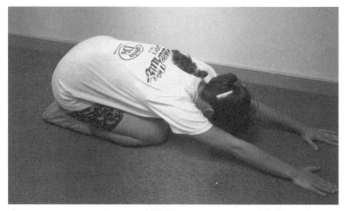

A

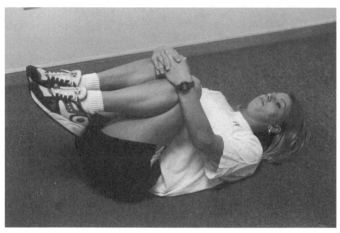

B

Figure 6A-15 The stretches depicted in this series of figures are commonly used stretches for the lumbar erector spinae, but many variations exist.

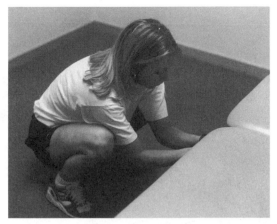

C

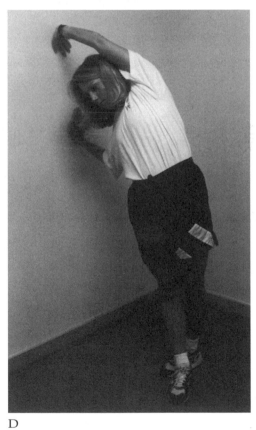

D

Figure 6A-15 *Continued*

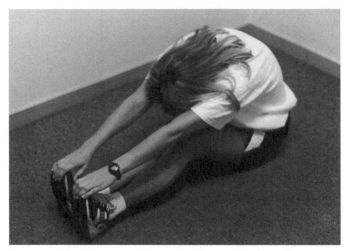

E

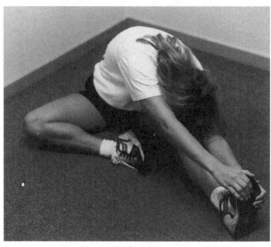

F

Figure 6A-15 *Continued*

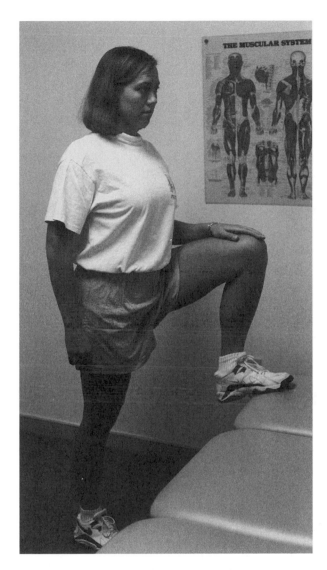

Figure 6A-16 To most effectively stretch the iliacus, the weightbearing lower extremity should be held in a neutral position, and the height of the surface on which the contralateral side is resting should allow the patient to feel a stretch and yet control the intensity of the stretch. As patients become more flexible, this surface will need to be raised. Although hip extension is encouraged, the lumbar spine should generally be kept in a neutral position.

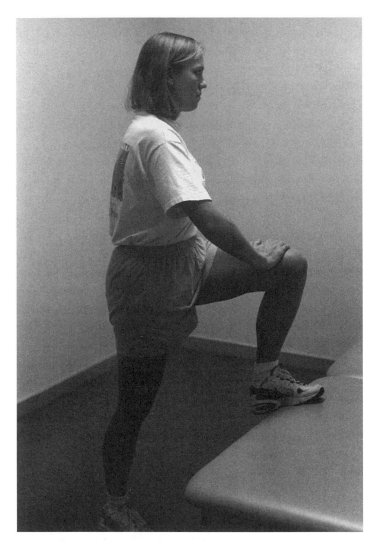

Figure 6A-17 The emphasis for this stretch is on the psoas major. This is a more complicated stretch that requires the patient to extend the lumbar spine and rotate slightly away from the side being stretched.

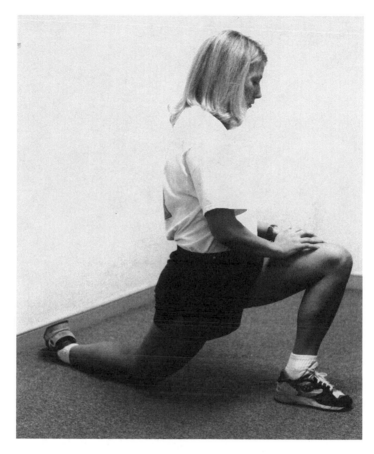

Figure 6A-18 This position generally stretches the proximal rectus femoris and can be used to stretch the iliacus and psoas major. This generally is a more complicated stretch and is not as easily mastered by most patients. If greater stretching on the rectus femoris is desired, the addition of greater knee flexion is necessary.

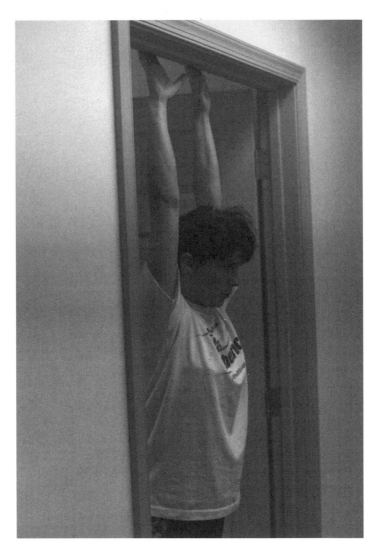

Figure 6A-19 To stretch the rectus abdominis, the patient is encouraged to gently distend the abdomen if additional stimulus is needed after elevating the ribs, anteriorly rotating the pelvis, and extending the lumbar spine.

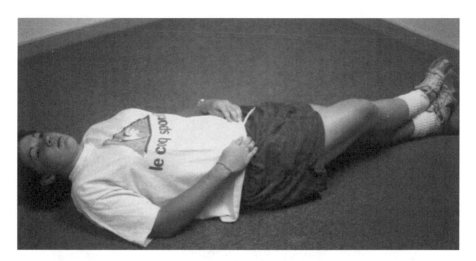

Figure 6A-20 To best stretch the hip abductors, the patient must keep the involved lower extremity in a neutral position with the knee slightly flexed.

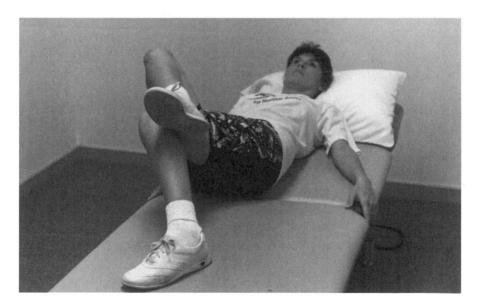

Figure 6A-21 The stretching of the hip abductors depicted in this figure must be performed with limited rotation of the pelvis and lumbar spine.

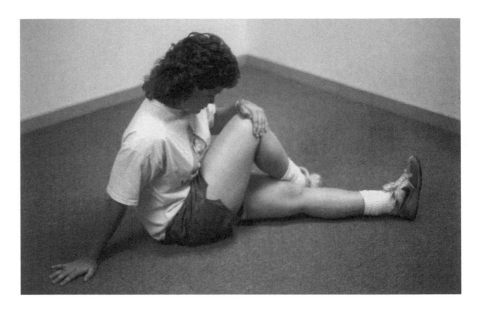

Figure 6A-22 There are multiple variations of this stretch for the hip abductors. The stretch depicted demonstrates what is generally considered to be the most difficult position. This is not, however, always the most effective stretch for the hip abductors.

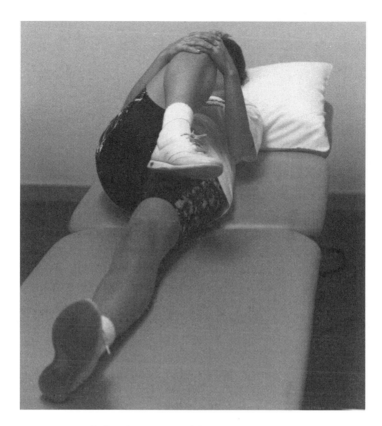

Figure 6A-23 A stretch for the proximal hip external rotators.

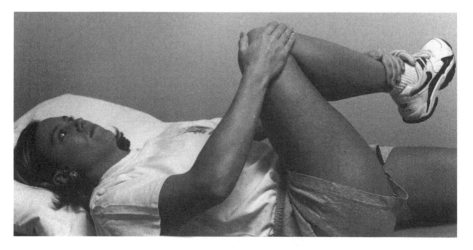

Figure 6A-24 This stretch emphasizes the distal hip external rotators with more hip flexion and relatively less internal rotation.

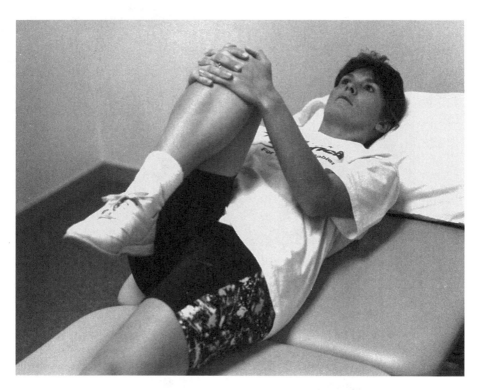

Figure 6A-25 This stretch is one of many possible for the hip extensors.

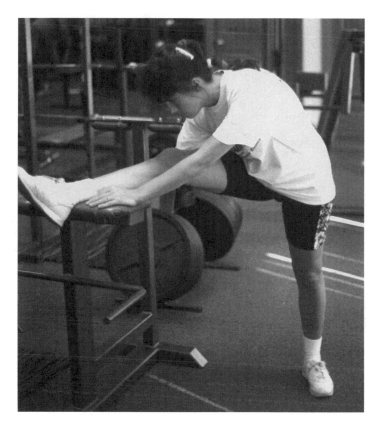

Figure 6A-26 In stretching the medial hamstrings, the contralateral limb is externally rotated in varying amounts to achieve a stretch in the desired location.

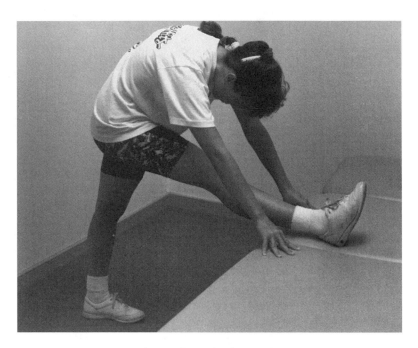

Figure 6A-27 One means of stretching the biceps femoris in which the contralateral lower extremity is kept in a relatively internally rotated position.

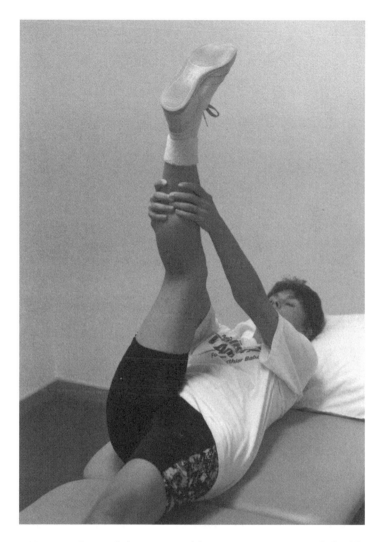

Figure 6A-28 Stretching of the proximal hamstrings is accomplished by allowing some knee flexion while requiring greater hip flexion.

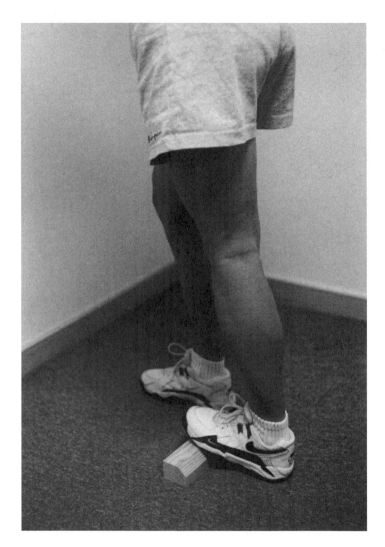

Figure 6A-29 The gastrocnemius is stretched by maintaining the ipsilateral lower extremity in a neutral position with the knee fully extended. A more advanced stretch uses an elevated surface under the metatarsal heads, as depicted here.

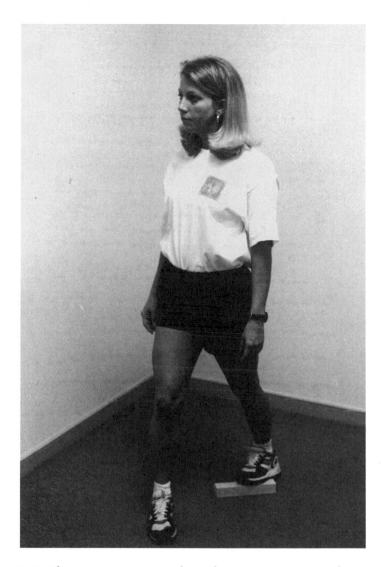

Figure 6A-30 This variation on stretching the gastrocnemius emphasizes the lateral and proximal fibers of the gastrocnemius by rotating the trunk and pelvis away from the side being stretched, leaving the tibia in an externally rotated position relative to the femur.

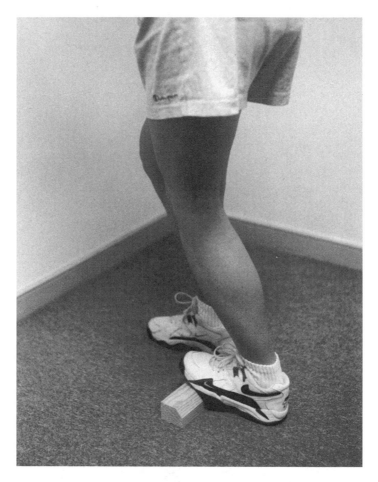

Figure 6A-31 To successfully stretch the soleus, the foot must be maintained in a neutral position, which is most easily enhanced by elevating the forefoot.

CHART # _____

O S PT A ORTHOPEDIC AND SPORTS PHYSICAL THERAPY ASSOCIATES, INC.

NAME _____ AGE _____ TELEPHONE_____

DATE STARTED _____ ADDRESS _____ MALE _____ FEMALE _____ WT. _____ HT. _____

LEGS	STANDING CALF RAISE	WT																							
		REP																							
		SET																							
	LEG CURL	WT																							
		REP																							
		SET																							
	LEG EXTENSIONS	WT																							
		REP																							
		SET																							
	SQUATS	WT																							
		REP																							
		SET																							
BACK	SEATED ROWS	WT																							
		REP																							
		SET																							
	PULL DOWNS	WT																							
		REP																							
		SET																							
	HYPER-EXTENSIONS	WT																							
		REP																							
		SET																							
	DEADLIFTS	WT																							
		REP																							
		SET																							
ABDOMINALS	SIT-UPS [CRUNCHES/BOARD]	WT																							
		REP																							
		SET																							
	LATERAL TRUNK BENDS	WT																							
		REP																							
		SET																							
CHEST	FLAT BENCH PRESS [BAR/DB]	WT																							
		REP																							
		SET																							
	INCLINE PRESS [BAR/DB]	WT																							
		REP																							
		SET																							
	DECLINE PRESS	WT																							
		REP																							
		SET																							

A

Figure 6A-32 (A) Normal patient identification information is recorded on the front of the patient's gym chart. Each day the patient's exercises are recorded along with the number of sets and repetitions and the amount of weights used for each exercise. Specific notations can be made on any day for any exercise regarding information pertinent to the patient's condition or the patient's experience with that specific exercise.

SHOULDERS	LATERAL RAISE [MACHINE/DB]	WT																													
		REP																													
		SET																													
	SHRUGS	WT																													
		REP																													
		SET																													
	OVERHEAD PRESS [DAR/DB]	WT																													
		REP																													
		SET																													
TRICEPS	TRICEP PRESS-DOWNS	WT																													
		REP																													
		SET																													
	CLOSE GRIP BENCH	WT																													
		REP																													
		SET																													
	TRICEP DB EXTENSION	WT																													
		REP																													
		SET																													
BICEPS	BB/DB CURLS [SEATED/ STANDING]	WT																													
		REP																													
		SET																													
	ISOLATION CURLS DB	WT																													
		REP																													
		SET																													
FOREARM	WRIST CURLS	WT																													
		REP																													
		SET																													
	WRIST EXTENSIONS	WT																													
		REP																													
		SET																													
		WT																													
		REP																													
		SET																													
		WT																													
		REP																													
		SET																													
		WT																													
		REP																													
		SET																													

B

Figure 6A-32 *Continued* (B) Several spaces are left blank on the back of the patient's gym chart for the addition of exercises not listed. (BB = barbell; DB = dumbbell; REP = repetitions; WT = weight.)

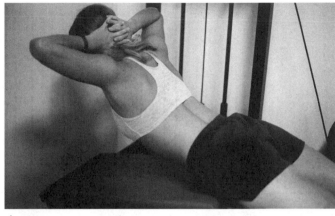

A

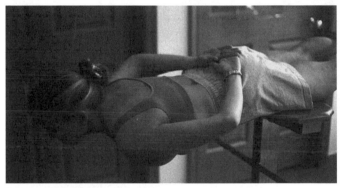

B

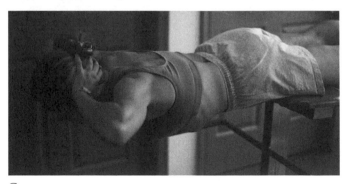

C

Figure 6A-33 (A) Hyperextensions performed with the patient's hands behind the neck are the first progression of this exercise. (B) Roman chair hyperextensions with the patient's hands behind the back are started once the patient has successfully completed two sets of 30 repetitions per set as shown in (A). (C) Roman chair hyperextensions are progressed by having the patient place the hands behind the neck.

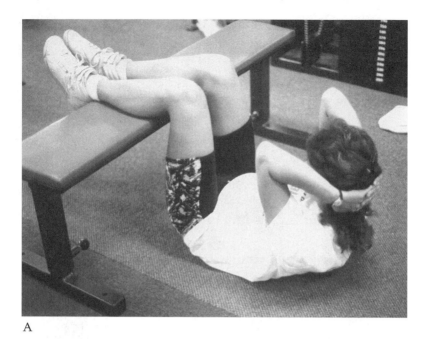

A

Figure 6A-34 (A) Crunches are perhaps the most common exercise for the rectus abdominis, as shown here. (B) This exercise can be supplemented by performing oblique crunches, which emphasize the internal and external obliques. When performing oblique crunches, the patient should be instructed not to rotate the cervical spine or to flex the cervical spine throughout the range. An attempt should be made to bring the elbow to the opposite knee for each repetition, which will ensure that roughly the same intensity of contraction is being performed with each repetition.

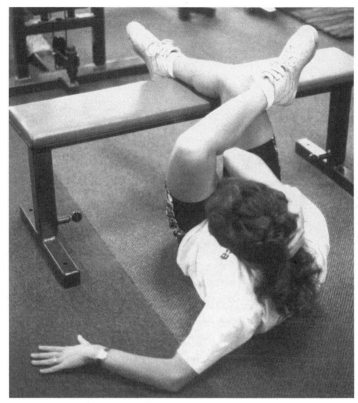

B

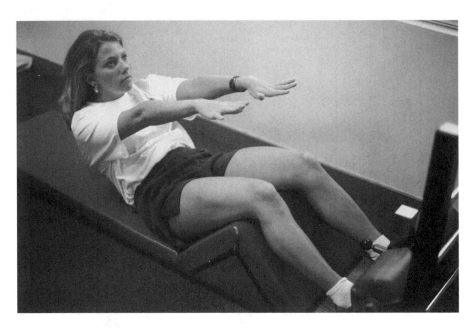

Figure 6A-35 The key elements in performing full-range sit-ups safely are to maintain a flattened lordosis at the beginning of the activity and when returning to a supine position. By starting the activity on a flat surface with the hands reaching forward and the cervical spine stabilized by maintaining a single position throughout the range, this exercise can be performed safely. Each repetition should be performed slowly and with considerable supervision to avoid the possibility of injury.

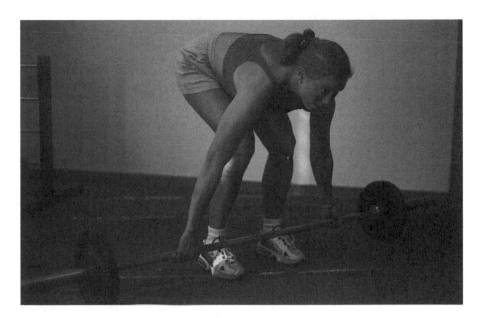

Figure 6A-36 Conventional dead lifts are performed by holding onto the bar so that the hands are placed wider than the feet. At all times, the bar is kept very close to the lower extremities (almost dragging it along the legs), the lumbar spine is in a neutral to slightly extended position, and the cervical spine is in some extension. When returning to an erect position, the legs initiate the lift but the erectors spinae complete the lift.

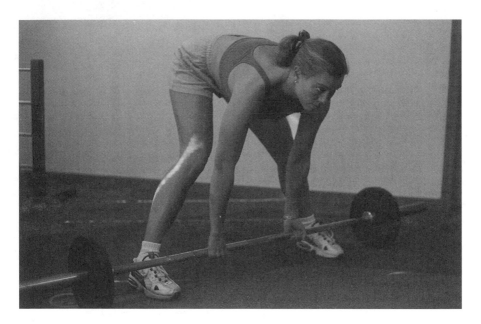

Figure 6A-37 This style of dead lifting is commonly referred to as the *sumo* style. The hands are placed on the bar between the knees, which allows the bar to be kept even closer to the body's center of gravity. The same principles for lifting apply as for the conventional method.

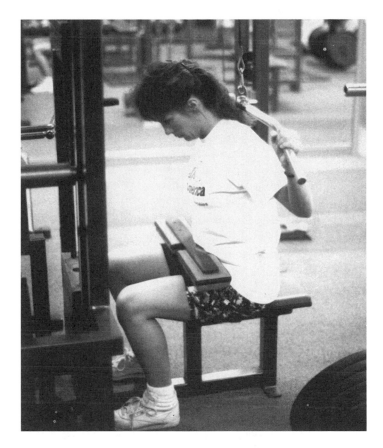

Figure 6A-38 Seated pull-downs can be performed with the bar either anterior or posterior to the cervical spine.

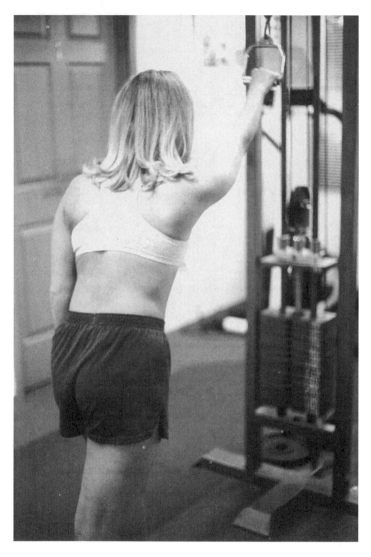

Figure 6A-39 Straight arm cable pull-downs are an effective way to isolate the latissimus dorsi unilaterally.

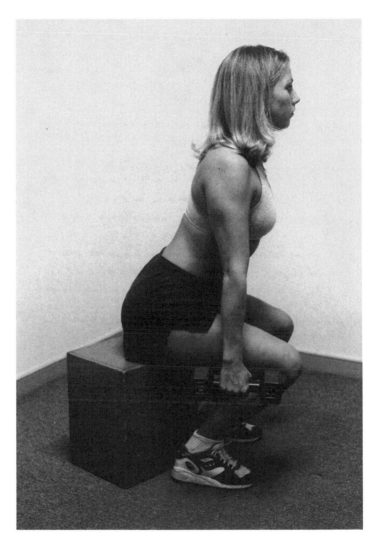

Figure 6A-40 Dumbbell squats are a complex activity involving multiple muscle groups and some co-contraction of the abdominals and erector spinae. Patients should perform the movement as if they were sitting down by maintaining a normal lumbar lordosis throughout the movement. The dumbbells should not be brought forward. Assuming there are no contraindications for this activity because of knee problems or some other condition, squats are an excellent way to pattern a movement that is important when performing normal lifting activities, either around the house or at work.

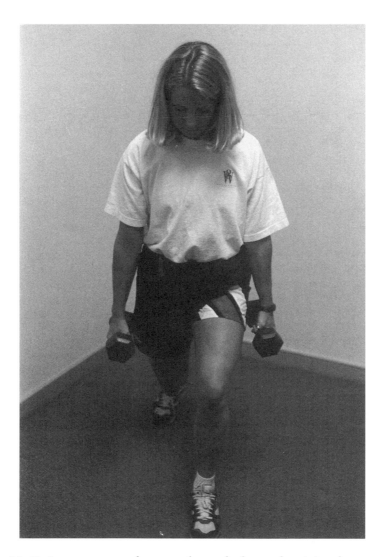

Figure 6A-41 Lunges are another complex and advanced activity that requires co-contraction of the abdominals and extensors, thus stabilizing the trunk while the lower extremities are moving. The activity is typically performed so that the knee on the leading lower extremity ultimately is flexed to approximately 90 degrees.

7

Postoperative Lumbar Rehabilitation

Brian P. D'Orazio, Caroline Tritsch,
Shane A. Vath, and
Marshall A. Rennie

History of Lumbar Surgery

Contemporary lumbar surgery can trace its origins to the early 1930s, when Mixter and Barr first published evidence directly linking low back pain (LBP) with lumbar intervertebral disc herniations.[1] Although other investigators recognized intervertebral disc lesions, they often viewed these lesions as tumors, classified as "chondromata." Mixter and Barr described disc lesions as ruptures, with laminectomy being the surgery of choice to expose and remove the ruptured material. This ground-breaking work led to an eventual proliferation of lumbar disc surgery, with a nearly universal assumption that LBP was inextricably linked to the intervertebral disc. In a discussion at the end of the paper by Mixter and Barr, Mixter introduced the concept of instability, stating that, "fusion should be combined with operation where there is any question of an unstable spine and I believe that a ruptured disc may be unstable." This theory of intervertebral disc disorders as the cause of LBP gradually usurped the theory that back pain was the result of arthritis generated by focal infections typically located in teeth, tonsils, and adenoids.[2]

In the 1970s and 1980s, evidence mounted regarding the failure of lumbar surgery to solve back pain. Interestingly, this occurred at a time when diagnostic imaging devices became available that improved intervertebral disc examination.

Current research indicates that back surgery rates in the United States are at least 40% higher than in any other country. The likelihood of someone undergoing back surgery in the United States is five times greater than in England or Scotland, with the surgery rate positively correlated with the numbers of surgeons in a given population. This led researchers to question whether Americans are subject to too much surgery or whether citizens of other countries are denied appropriate treatment.[3]

With evidence mounting that pathologic conditions of the disc often do not correlate with complaints of LBP, the segmental instability theory has gradually become the focus of both conservative and surgical corrective measures.[4-6] Despite controversy in identification of instability or its relationship to pain, surgical and dynamic lumbar stabilization have proliferated. Results from surgical stabilizations vary greatly, with consistent evidence of poorer outcomes among patients with a pseudarthrosis. To reduce the pseudarthrosis rate, a variety of treatment options have been introduced, including repeat surgery. Yet research clearly indicates the chances of surgical success diminish greatly after repeat surgery, with psychosocial factors proving to be better predictors of success than physical factors. Consequent to these controversies, selection criteria for surgical candidates is being established, with surgeons making efforts to restrain their patients' "irrational exuberance" over the promise that surgery is a cure.[7,8]

Research has yet to conclude the best time at which to begin rehabilitation or how rehabilitation is best delivered among specific subcategories of postoperative lumbar patients. The literature strongly supports the need for high-intensity exercise programs of long duration to achieve maximum medical improvement among postoperative lumbar patients.[9-15] This opposes current dogma, mostly from insurance companies, purporting that adequate outcomes are achieved with little postsurgical rehabilitation.

The remainder of this chapter begins with a discussion of basic surgical techniques followed by outcomes and rehabilitation techniques for these surgical procedures. The rehabilitation guidelines are broad, with protocols based on research and clinical experience. Support for the treatment protocols comes from both clinical and basic science research on tissue healing and physiologic responses to trauma.

Types of Surgical Procedures

Evaluating the need and type of rehabilitation necessary for a patient who has undergone lumbar surgery begins by understanding the various surgical approaches to pathologic conditions of the spine. Physical therapists should become familiar with the various surgical procedures, using the operative notes to confirm surgical findings.

Table 7-1 summarizes the common operative approaches to pathologic conditions of the lumbar spine. Most are intended to address disc disease or injury. Although some studies exist comparing the techniques, there is still

Table 7-1 Common Decompressive Surgical Procedures

Surgery type	Procedure
Percutaneous discectomy	A specialized needle is used to remove only the herniated portion of a disc.
Microdiscectomy	A surgical microscope is used to aid a minimal incision technique that removes the herniated portions of the disc with the option of also removing intradiscal material.
Foraminotomy	The intervertebral foramen is enlarged by removing part of the anterior facets, called a subarticular fenestration, removing protruding osteophytes, and removing any surrounding osseous structure that reduces foraminal size.
Laminotomy	To gain greater access to the intervertebral disc, part of the laminae is excised, typically in combination with a foraminotomy.
Hemilaminectomy	This is achieved with the unilateral excision of the vertebral laminae.
Laminectomy	This surgery involves bilateral removal of the vertebral laminae including the spinous process.
Internal laminoplasty	The spinal canal is enlarged internally by an undercutting facetectomy performed through an opening created by removing the spinous process.

widespread disagreement over which produces the best results. With percutaneous discectomy, only the herniated portion of the disc is removed. When partial discectomy is combined with the other surgical procedures, typically sequestered portions of the disc and significant intradiscal material are removed.

A visual representation of bone removal is shown in Figure 7-1. Young et al. reported that by removing the medial third of each facet, an ample surgical window is created through which neural tissue is decompressed and disc material can be removed.[16]

Many lumbar procedures can be performed on an outpatient basis, such as a unilateral nerve root decompression for foraminal stenosis.[17] Combinations of pathologic conditions, such as a foraminal stenosis complicated by a far lateral disc herniation, typically require more surgery, which is usually performed on an in-patient basis.[18] Additionally, there are varied approaches to surgical correction of similar pathologic entities. Physical therapists

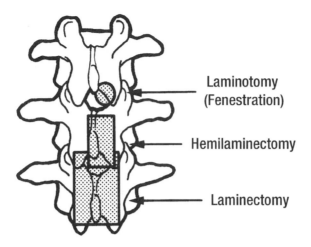

Figure 7-1 Typical osseous windows created by the specified surgical procedures. (Reprinted with permission from RC Childs, GBJ Andersson. Rehabilitation after Back Surgery. In BP D'Orazio [ed], Back Pain Rehabilitation. Boston: Andover Medical Publishers, 1993;72.)

should not assume, for example, that a far lateral disc herniation will be managed in a specific fashion. Epstein pointed out that in the management of far lateral discs, total facetectomy provides the best exposure but increases the risk of instability, whereas laminotomy with medial facetectomy exposes the lateral and subarticular recesses but visualization of the far lateral component is often inadequate.[19] Using an intertransverse approach offers excellent far lateral recess visualization but not medial intraforaminal exposure.[19] Figure 7-2 depicts some of the surgical procedures.

Table 7-2 lists common fusions and provides information regarding fusion procedures. As in many areas of musculoskeletal medicine, the technologic advances in fusion procedures precede research to validate the procedures. It is beyond the intent of this chapter to present more than basic details regarding fusions.

Physiologic Healing Response of Tissue

At least 14 types of human collagen have been identified; however, all mature scars are formed from type I collagen. During the last phase of healing, the scar matures to take on the physical characteristics of the tissue it replaces. This transition is in response to internal and external influ-

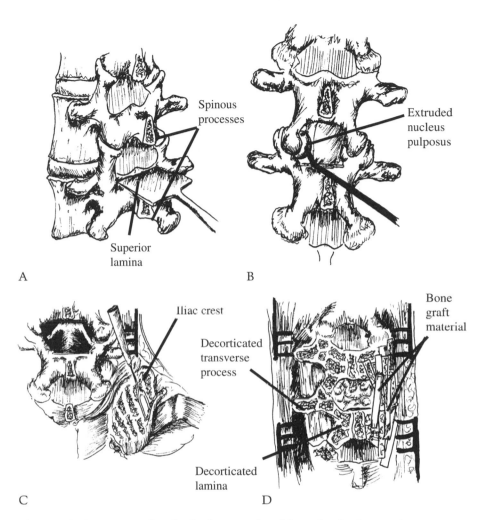

Figure 7-2 Decompression for both central and lateral spinal stenosis.
(A) Removal of the spinous process and resection of the superior portion of the lamina. (B) Removal of the extruded nucleus pulposus as well as the enlarging of any laminar defect. (C) When fusion is required, bone is harvested from the ilium, posteriorly. (D) Fusion is accomplished with the decortication of the dorsal surfaces of the laminae, transverse processes, and upper sacrum with bone graft material placed across the lateral gutters on both sides. (Illustrated by Jeff Telemeco.)

Table 7-2 Common Surgical Fusion Procedures

Surgery type	Procedure
Noninstrumented posterolateral fusion	Bone grafts from the iliac crest are used to fuse the facets, pars interarticularis, and the adjoining transverse processes.
Instrumented posterolateral fusion	Posterolateral bone fusion is used with the addition of instrumentation to immobilize the segment or segments being fused. Current techniques usually use rigid instrumentation.
Noninstrumented anterior interbody fusion	Once the disc is removed, bone blocks are placed across the disc space.
Instrumented anterior interbody fusion	Once the bony blocks have been placed across the disc space, hardware is used to increase stability, usually when more than one disc level is performed.

Source: Adapted from AH Crenshaw (ed). Campbell's Operative Orthopaedics (8th ed). Baltimore: Mosby–Year Book, 1992;3583.

ences, which cause scar differentiation.[20] Underlying disease processes such as diabetes, peripheral vascular disease, hypertension, congestive heart failure, and poor nutritional status can lead to delayed healing.[20,21] Smoking has a negative effect on bone healing and is associated with increased rates of pseudarthrosis.[21] Because of the overwhelming number of variables that influence tissue healing, temporal changes in healing rates are fluid, even within a single wound.[20]

Tissue healing is a three-phase dynamic process that begins at wound closure and continues well after the incision is healed (Table 7-3). The inflammatory phase lasts 3–4 days and is the body's initial response to the surgical trauma. The immediate release of vasoactive substances causes increased vascular dilation and permeability. A cascade of events leads to the release of macrophages, which aid in the removal of necrotic tissue and byproducts caused by the surgical trauma.[20,21] Insufficient inflammation slows healing, whereas aggressive inflammation results in excessive scar production.[20] Mechanical stress applied to the incised area leads to increased inflammation. Treatment should consist of rest, ice, elevation, and compression of the involved area; the cardiovascular system should be stressed to decrease the negative effects of postoperative immobilization. Early ambulation decreases use of postoperative pain medication.[21]

The collagen repair phase peaks approximately 7–10 days postoperatively and slows by the end of the second week. At the end of this phase, the wound

Table 7-3 Normal Tissue Healing

Healing phase	Time from surgery	Physiologic response	Therapeutic goals
Inflammation	Wound closure to day 4	Vascular dilation Macrophages	Control inflammation and edema
Repair	Days 7–14	Capillary ingrowth Collagen production	Edema management Progressive mobilization
Maturation	Day 14–1 year	Collagen maturation	Restore full motion Progressive resistive exercise

has amassed the greatest amount of collagen; however, these fibers are poorly arranged, immature, and lack the tensile strength of mature scar.[20,21]

The maturation phase starts at 14 days and lasts from 6 months to 1 year. The application of tension through exercise results in an increase in tensile strength, whereas immobilization and stress deprivation result in a loss of normal collagen alignment and decreased tensile strength.[20,21]

Muscle and Nerve

Muscle Atrophy

Low back surgery creates a varied amount of damage to the soft tissues and bone of the lumbar spine. To preserve the integrity of the erector spinae, they are dissected off the spinous processes rather than incising across the erector spinae, which ultimately weakens the integrity of the muscle unit. Muscle innervation is also spared with this technique, although, "electromyographic [EMG] studies of back muscles after surgery typically show denervation potentials for a long time."[21]

Lumbosacral nerve retraction is common in many lumbar surgical procedures. Nerve root blood flow decreases with increasing retraction pressure, sometimes leading to myotomal and dermatomal disturbances.[22] Sihvonen and colleagues studied paraspinal muscles in successful and failed laminectomies 2–5 years after surgery.[23] The failed group displayed abnormal denervation potentials on EMG studies and atrophy on computed tomographic (CT) scan.[23] Atrophy, found at the operative level, was secondary to nerve or muscle injury caused by either the surgical approach or disuse. Atrophy found at the inoperative levels was most likely caused by disuse.[23] Rantanen et al. found "that both inactivity and axonal injury contribute to the selective type II atrophy and inner structure changes in disc patients' multifidus muscle. These pathologic structural changes correlated well with clinical outcome, and most importantly they are reversible and can be diminished by adequate therapy."[15] Surgical techniques should incorporate intermittent release of retraction throughout the procedure to help minimize nerve root injury during posterior lumbar surgery.[15,22]

Fibrosis of Nerve

Lumbar disc surgery commonly leads to epidural or radicular scarring.[24-26] Jensen reported that 88% of patients presented with dural radicular scar tissue within 3 months after surgery.[26] Although scarring of the nerves is common, research indicates there is no correlation between diagnostic imaging findings of neural fibrosis and reports of symptoms.[24,26] Furthermore, Annertz et al.[24] found that among eight patients who underwent surgery to remove scar tissue, all initially experienced some relief of sciatica; however, six of the eight reported their symptoms returned and intensified within 12 months after surgery. The authors recommended that repeat decompressive surgery for epidural fibrosis "should be refrained from if other morphological causes of compression can be excluded."[24]

Sources of Nerve Pain

Many mechanisms of radicular pain have been proposed, including nerve root compression, fibrosis, motion segment instability, diabetic lumbar radiculopathy, and iatrogenic nerve palsy.[22,27-29] Human experiments have shown that only inflamed nerve roots that are compressed or elongated can elicit radicular pain, yet studies have demonstrated that 20–30% of subjects without a history of pain demonstrate evidence of compressed nerve roots on diagnostic imaging.[28] Another proposed mechanism for radicular pain is instability following a laminectomy and partial discectomy. Instability is believed to cause greater tension on the nerve root, leading to nerve root pain. Cadaveric studies, however, demonstrate equal nerve root motion with straight leg raising when comparing multilevel laminectomies with and without rigid stabilization.[27] The most recent hypothesis for the cause of radicular pain is summarized in Figure 7-3.

Bone Healing and Pain

Bone used in spinal fusions is typically obtained via autogenous grafts from the iliac crest. Some sources indicate the need for postoperative immobilization via a body cast or thoracolumbar orthosis for varying times ranging from 2 months to (typically) 6 months.[30] Full fusion consolidation

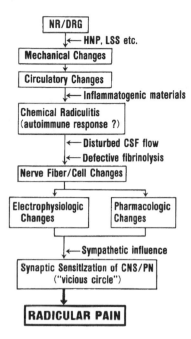

Figure 7-3 Hypothesis for the pathomechanism of radicular pain. (NR = nerve root; DRG = dorsal root ganglion; HNP = herniated nucleus pulposus; LSS = lumbar spinal stenosis; CSF = cerebrospinal fluid; CNS = central nervous system; PN = peripheral nerve.) Hasue noted that "[t]hese morphologic, circulatory, biomechanical, pathologic, electrophysiologic, and pharmacologic changes may finally result in sensitization of both the central and peripheral nervous systems, causing radicular pain."[28] (Reprinted with permission from M Hasue. Pain and the nerve root: an interdisciplinary approach. Spine 1993;18:2053.)

commonly requires 12 months, during which time it is typical for a patient to complain of donor site pain along the iliac crest and sensory deficits in the same region.[21,30] In addition to bone healing, there is also the issue of donor site pain and sensation deficits. Sensory deficits of the donor site are reported to be twice as high when a separate lateral incision is used for harvesting bone versus use of the midline incision. Extending the incision laterally places the cluneal nerves at risk of transection. Donor site pain, however, is apparently not influenced by the harvesting of bone via the primary midline incision versus a separate lateral incision. Psychosocial elements are thought to play a role in the perpetuation of chronic donor site pain, because patients undergoing spinal reconstructive procedures report twice the incidence of donor site pain as patients undergoing surgery for spinal trauma.[31]

Mechanical Properties and Healing of the Intervertebral Disc

Studies involving lumbar disc herniations treated nonsurgically have demonstrated that a decrease in size of the herniation will occur over time. The amount of time and the specific mechanism of disc resorption have not been clearly identified.[6,32] Also lacking in research is the specific physiologic healing response of an injured lumbar intervertebral disc. It is well known that lumbar intradiscal pressure increases are greater with flexion and lateral bending than with extension and torsional movements of the same magnitude. Healthy lumbar discs are able to resist substantial axial compressive loads with cartilaginous end plate and bony fracture occurring without disc rupture.[33–36] Using an in vitro disc model, Gordon et al. concluded that disc prolapse occurs "when the appropriate combination of flexion, rotation and compression operate over an adequate length of time."[37] Unfortunately, the question of how much force a surgically treated disc can take without reinjury has not been examined.

Conditions Requiring Surgery: Outcomes and Rehabilitation

Disc lesions, spinal stenosis, and vertebral instability are the three most common conditions that sometimes require surgical management. This section limits discussion to these three general conditions, the surgical procedures typically performed, and postoperative rehabilitation.

Disc Lesions

Table 7-4 defines common disc lesions that are treated surgically. In this table, the term *herniation* has been divided into two descriptors: protrusion and extrusion. This classification was proposed to improve the uniformity of magnetic resonance imaging (MRI) observations by radiologists. The authors observed that extrusions were infrequent in asymptomatic patients, whereas protrusions and disc bulges are commonly observed in an asymptomatic population. Surgery on disc protrusions and bulges may be one reason for lowered success rates among spinal surgeons, because a direct correlation between these entities and the patient's pain is more difficult to establish.[38]

Outcomes

Long believed that the failed back surgery syndrome is multidimensional.[7] Rehabilitation failure may be the result of structural abnormalities, psychosocial issues, or a combination of both factors. Even when a lesion

Table 7-4 Disc Lesion Classifications

Type of lesion	Definition
Bulge	The annulus of the intervertebral disc circumferentially extending beyond the plane of the vertebral end plates
Protrusion	An asymmetric extension of the intervertebral disc with the base of the extension being wider than the distal portion of the extension
Extrusion	The extended fragment is wider than its connection to the intervertebral disc

Source: Adapted from M Brant-Zawadzki, M Jensen. Imaging corner spinal nomenclature. Spine 1995;20:388.

is found that appears to correlate with the patient's symptoms, patients should still attempt rehabilitation to regain function. *Patients are best treated using a comprehensive program that addresses the complex psychosocial issues.*[7,39]

Determining outcomes after lumbar disc surgery is complicated by multiple variables, including absence of objective outcome measures, lack of randomization, inclusion of multiple surgical techniques, varying degrees of psychosocial factors, and when and on whom to perform surgery. Various lumbar surgery techniques are lumped together, which also leads to increased variability in outcomes. Measurements of postsurgical outcomes are often poorly defined and subjective. Last, because of the serious nature of lumbar disc surgery, it is not appropriate to randomly assign patients to a surgical versus nonsurgical treatment group.[40,41]

Postacchini noted that *"many operations for lumbar disc herniation could probably be avoided if energetic conservative management was continued for longer periods before surgery was considered."*[41] It has been observed that herniations decrease in size or disappear; however, the probability and length of time for this process to occur is unknown.[41,42] There is not a strong correlation between a patient's symptoms and the presence or degree of disc herniation.[25] In patients with radiculitis, the optimal length of time to continue conservative treatment is unknown.[41]

Patients with sciatica generally improve regardless of the type of treatment. At 1 year after surgery, patients treated surgically reported better symptomatic improvement than nonsurgically treated patients.[40] This did not result in substantial differences in either employment or workers' compensation status.[40] After 4 years, patients with and without surgery fared about equally.[43] For patients who have minor symptoms, surgical intervention appears to have minimal benefits.[40] Because surgery does appear to more rapidly resolve symptoms, patients who require a rapid resolution of symptoms or who have more severe pain should be considered as candidates for disc surgery.[41]

Rehabilitation After Disc Surgery

Manniche stated that "*in the future it would be ideal if all discus operated patients had the opportunity to undergo postoperative supervised training. Both the psychological support as well as the physical improvements from training would most likely reduce the number of patients who lose considerable work capabilities.*"[11] Furthermore, Manniche and others have concluded that not only is rehabilitation necessary after surgery, but exercise intensity also is important.[9–12,14,15] Although some patients seem to do well after lumbar disc surgery, many will experience significantly reduced physical capabilities and unnecessary pain in the absence of rehabilitation. Manniche reported this number to be approximately 25%.[11] A 25% morbidity rate is extremely high in terms of personal and societal cost. Consequently, all patients would benefit from a formalized program of postoperative rehabilitation.

Carragee et al. found that postoperative activity restrictions were unnecessary, and allowing patients to proceed without restrictions led to better outcomes.[44] Clinicians who unnecessarily restrict activities combined with the patients' fear of exacerbating symptoms by embarking on a rehabilitation program can limit outcomes. Patients must be told that exercise may transiently increase symptoms. Clinicians need to reinforce this information with considerable psychological and treatment support, especially during the first several weeks of rehabilitation, because symptom reduction may occur only after considerable strength gains are achieved.[11,13] Most contemporary lumbar disc surgical procedures do not destabilize the lumbar spine. Exercise programs, however, should allow for many variables, including the static and dynamic stability of the spine, the patient's physical condition, the patient's psychological response to both the pain and the surgery, physical impairments, age, osteoporosis, smoking, and other issues that clinicians encounter daily. Throughout this book, these variables have been discussed and the reader should reference those specific circumstances when making decisions about how to proceed with a patient's post-lumbar surgery rehabilitation program.

Temporal Considerations for Postoperative Rehabilitation

Patients should receive professional rehabilitation within 48 hours after surgery. During the first 24 hours, patients usually begin walking. Cryotherapy, appropriate pain medication, and adequate instructions on body mechanics are the main treatments during the first 7 days after most surgeries. Table 7-5 provides a chronology for rehabilitation after most lumbar surgery. The guidelines provided by Table 7-5 are intentionally general, allowing for individuality and innovation in the prescription of rehabilitation by physical therapists. For minimally invasive procedures, the time line can be moved forward by up to 1 week if the patient is recovering uneventfully and the surgeon is in agreement. Prescription of specific exercises can be adapted from those presented in Chapter 6.

Abdominal exercises should begin shortly after surgery. After 7 days, light, mostly isometric abdominal exercises can be performed. These can be progressed gradually for weeks 1 and 2 after surgery and then by week 3 and beyond, the abdominal exercise program should become rigorous and part of the patient's exercise prescription for life.

The initial strategy of "walking" in Table 7-5 starts the patient with several walks daily to tolerance. When patients reach 2 miles, they walk once daily, eventually progressing walking distances to 3 or 4 miles.

During the first 2 weeks, exercises that do not directly stretch the erector spinae can be performed. Because stretching of the hip extensors indirectly stretches the erector spinae, these stretches can be started about 7 days postoperatively, but by 6 weeks, they usually do not need to be continued. Hamstring stretching that minimally stresses the surgical site should be started soon after surgery and continued during the first 2 weeks. By the third week, hamstring exercises should be increased and should have a greater impact on the surgical site and the lumbar erector spinae.

Dynamic lumbar exercises are intended to improve control of movement as well as segmental function. By the ninth week, these movements are performed with great proficiency and are not continued, although some exercises to maintain intersegmental mobility may need to be performed beyond this time.

Given the data reported earlier in this chapter, rehabilitation of the lumbar erector spinae is probably the most important aspect of postoperative rehabilitation. The erector spinae will not strengthen to normal levels without an adequate stimulus. As a consequence, the postoperative rehabilitation protocol presented in Table 7-5 strongly emphasizes lumbar erector spinae rehabilitation and progresses the program beyond that prescribed by many clinicians. The use of extension exercises, progressed sequentially as noted in the previous chapter, leads to excellent outcomes, improving strength, range of motion, dynamic lumbar stabilization, and pain control.

The performance of dead lifts has remained controversial. If dead lifts are performed when indicated and with excellent form, the risk to patients is extremely low. The risk to patients in not performing this activity is

Table 7-5 Rehabilitation After Common Disc Surgical Procedures

Rehabilitation strategies	Time after surgery						
	0–7 days	1–2 weeks	3–6 weeks	6–9 weeks	9–12 weeks	12–16 weeks	16+ weeks
Education	■	■	■	■	■	■	■
Use of analgesics	■	■	■	■	■		
Cryotherapy	■	■	■				
Walking	■	■	■	■			
Hamstring stretching with minimal lumbar involvement	■	■	■				
Stretching of hip extensors		■	■				
Stretching of other muscles with minimal lumbar involvement	■	■	■				
Dynamic lumbar exercises for movement reintegration		■	■	■			
Abdominal exercises			■	■	■	■	■
Erector spinae stretching, progress stretching of other muscles			■	■	■	■	■
Upper extremity exercises			■	■	■	■	
Lower extremity exercises			■	■	■	■	
Exercise for the lumbar erector spinae		■	■	■	■	■	■
Progressive walking beyond 2 miles			■	■	■	■	
Functional activities and work simulation				■	■	■	
Exercise prescription for life						■	■

extremely high. This is the activity that most commonly causes acute exacerbations when performed in normal daily activities. Training patients to lift appropriately is essential in preventing future exacerbations. Adequately strengthening the erector spinae through this means is a prerequisite to allowing the patient to return to those types of activities. The combination of dead lifts and extension exercises adequately strengthens most portions of the lumbar erector spinae, thus stabilizing this region for normal activities. If dead lifts are progressed ahead of the other phases of rehabilitation, too much stress will be applied to the lower lumbar spine, thereby increasing the risk of injury. The physical therapist must appropriately sequence activities so as not to place the patient at risk from the rehabilitation program.

Patients who smoke, and especially those who smoke heavily, are more likely to suffer from disc degeneration, and clinically it seems that these patients are more easily injured in a rehabilitation program.[45–47] At our office, we strongly recommend that patients discontinue smoking and we progress this patient population somewhat slower than nonsmokers.

Table 7-5 takes rehabilitation to 16 weeks and beyond, although many patients will not require 16 weeks of formal rehabilitation. By the end of 16 weeks, patients should be well advanced in an exercise program and probably can perform the program independently. Functional activities and work simulation are usually performed during weeks 6–12. Most patients will return to work by the end of the twelfth week, although patients in jobs that require heavy labor may not be ready after 12 weeks.

The failure to prescribe adequate intensity to the patient's rehabilitation program leads to poorer outcomes.[9–11,14] Those patients returning to heavy manual labor tasks require a more intense program of rehabilitation than others. Even the most sedentary individual, however, routinely engages in fairly vigorous spinal activities such as routine work around the house or sexual intercourse, thus placing considerable demand on the trunk musculature. Furthermore, adequate rehabilitation of the spine often includes upper and lower extremity rehabilitation. Inadequate upper extremity strength may cause patients to rely more on their back for lifting. Adequate lower extremity function is essential in decreasing the demands placed on the lumbar spine. Although differences of opinion exist as to how we should lift objects, use of the lower extremities is necessary in most lifts. Many patients are unable to perform a squat without a weight, much less with a weight. As a result, an adequate lower extremity reconditioning program is essential.

For those patients with chronic pain, adequate psychological support should be provided, as stated previously. Many of these patients should be referred to a mental health professional. To do less is to provide inadequate care and compromise the final patient outcome. Because chronic pain has

Table 7-6 Classifications of Acquired Spinal Stenosis

Type	Location
Central	Central portion of the canal
Lateral recess	"Bordered laterally by the pedicle, posteriorly by the superior articular facet and anteriorly by the posterolateral surface of the vertebral body and the adjacent intervertebral disc"
Foraminal	Intervertebral foramen—that is, between the superior and inferior pedicles of adjoining vertebra
Far out	Between large L5 transverse process and the sacrum (mostly seen in spondylolisthesis)

Source: Adapted from AH Crenshaw (ed). Campbell's Operative Orthopaedics (8th ed). Baltimore: Mosby–Year Book, 1992;3836.

lifelong consequences for that individual, there can be no excuse to not make this referral.

Lumbar Spinal Stenosis: Outcomes and Rehabilitation

Spinal stenosis is a narrowing of the spinal canal centrally or laterally. When the narrowing is caused by fetal development, it is referred to as congenital stenosis. Acquired stenosis occurs as a result of degenerative changes. Classifications of acquired spinal stenosis are defined predominantly by the location of the degeneration changes (Table 7-6). One region whose name may be a bit deceptive is the lateral recess, which is actually located within the central canal.

Both congenital and acquired spinal stenosis clinically cause LBP, sciatica, and claudication symptoms. Surgery is an option to rid a patient of these symptoms by increasing the available space for the cauda equina or nerve roots via various forms of surgical decompression.

A simple explanation of why this narrowing induces symptoms was offered by Winston et al., who found decreased lumbar canal dimensions in patients who underwent surgery for lumbar radiculopathy compared with controls.[48] Thus, it requires only a small disc protrusion or structural abnormality to impinge the nerve.[48] The central spinal canal gradually narrows, with the canal diameter at L1 being relatively larger than the canal diameter at L5.[49] This is one explanation for the higher incidence of nerve root involvement in the more caudal nerves.[50]

Another possible explanation of cauda equina symptoms was offered by Takahashi et al., who found a correlation between increased epidural pressure and posture.[51] Epidural pressure at stenotic levels was low in recumbency and sitting and relatively high in standing. In combination with the fact that extension typically reduces the canal diameter, postural changes that increase pressure may induce compression of nerve roots or the cauda equina, thus producing radicular symptoms.

The comparison of surgical and nonsurgical management of spinal stenosis has been studied sparsely. Atlas et al. found that surgically treated patients showed more improvement than nonsurgically treated patients at 1 year.[52] Later, in a time frame not specified by the authors, the two groups were not statistically different.[52] Johnsson et al. studied surgical versus conservative treatment with a 2–3 year follow-up and found that the level of pain did not differ significantly between the two groups and both reported an increase in walking capacity.[53] The study concluded that the patients who declined surgery did well for at least 2–3 years without obvious deterioration, and neurophysiologic deterioration was not prevented by surgery. When stenosis was treated with laminectomy, patients continued improving over time and few required additional surgery.[54]

Far lateral recesses stenosis, described previously, can be caused by congenital lumbosacral anomalies such as a transition vertebra. Nerve roots can be compressed between the transverse processes of the last formed vertebral level and either the sacrum or ilium (Figure 7-4). This can also be created by other factors, such as loss of intervertebral disc height.[55]

Studies on patient satisfaction after spinal stenosis surgery indicate that patient selection is important. Factors leading to good postsurgical outcomes include no prior surgical intervention; no comorbidity of diabetes, hip arthrosis, preoperative fractures of the lumbar spine, or multiple medical problems; good preoperative functional status; and a predominance of leg symptoms.[56,57] This confirms the widely held belief that decompressive spinal surgery is generally most effective in those patients with lower extremity symptoms. This can be objectively shown by an increase in treadmill walking tolerance after laminectomy secondary to a decrease in intermittent neurogenic claudication symptoms.[58] Symptoms are relieved by cessation of ambulation and typically forward bending. Forward bending increases the sagittal diameter of the spinal canal, which conversely usually decreases with extension of the vertebral column (Figure 7-5). A small percentage of patients exhibit an increase in vertebral canal diameter with extension.[59]

Nonsurgical approaches for spinal stenosis include epidural injections, anti-inflammatory medications, and specific rehabilitation procedures.

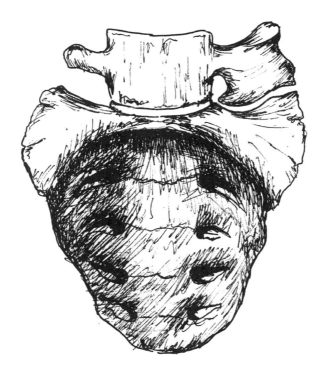

Figure 7-4 Sacralization of the fifth lumbar vertebrae. (Illustrated by Jeff Telemeco.)

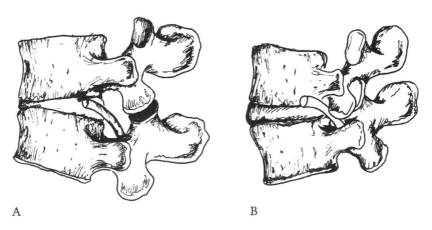

A   B

Figure 7-5 Effects of lumbar hyperlordosis and flexion on spinal nerve roots. (A) Lumbar spine in flexion. (B) Lumbar spine in hyperextension. (Illustrated by Jeff Telemeco.)

Therapeutic epidural injections using corticosteroids temporarily reduce inflammation and local edema, which is sometimes helpful to the patient's rehabilitation program.

Rehabilitation must consider posture as a variable requiring treatment. Because flexion is desired to open the spinal canal, teaching the patient to reduce lordosis when recumbent, standing, and sitting helps reduce symptoms. Factors that may increase lordosis should be addressed, such as reduced length of the iliacus, which anteriorly tilts the pelvis, sitting in a seat that is too high, walking in shoes with heels, decreased flexibility of the ankle plantar flexors, and, at least theoretically, decreased muscle length of the lumbar erector spinae. An increase in thoracic kyphosis may also cause the patient to compensate by increasing lumbar lordosis, which may increase symptoms. An increase in thoracic kyphosis, however, may also decrease the lordosis, and this must be evaluated on an individual basis.

Low back strengthening is also necessary after surgery. Muscle atrophy from disuse secondary to pain or bed rest as well as dorsal rami lesions after surgical procedures can lead to prolonged pain. Strengthening of the erector spinae was discussed in Chapter 6. Presumably, the surgery has eliminated the decrease in spinal canal diameter, therefore allowing for spinal extension. If stenosis at other levels still prevents extension of the lumbar spine, a variety of exercises are available for the erector spinae that do not cause significant extension of the lumbar spine. Rehabilitation may differ according to the specific surgical procedure for spinal stenosis, such as fusion versus a laminotomy. Additionally, spinal stenosis patients often have lower extremity symptoms caused by nerve root compression. Once the nerve roots have been decompressed surgically, lower extremity weakness may persist, thus necessitating a comprehensive lower extremity reconditioning program. All individuals will not be rehabilitated at the same rate secondary to multiple confounding factors, such as age, cardiovascular status, neurologic damage, and other medical problems.

Lumbar Instability and Surgical Fusion

Fusion

Deyo et al. reported that from 1979 through 1987 spinal fusion was the fastest growing technique for spinal surgery, increasing at a rate of approximately 200%.[60] Spinal fusion is performed for many reasons, some better understood than others. In the case of spinal stenosis, fusion is used when the surgeon believes a laminectomy will destabilize the spine. Fusion is commonly used for spondylolisthesis, typically with radiographic evidence of vertebral instability and a vertebral slip of 50% or greater. Fusion is

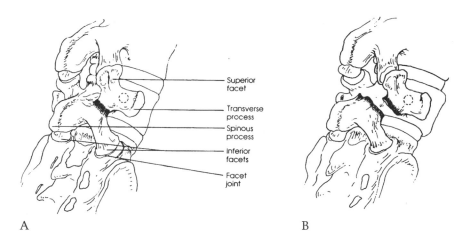

Labels (left illustration A):
- Superior facet
- Transverse process
- Spinous process
- Inferior facets
- Facet joint

A   B

Figure 7-6 (A) Spondylolysis and (B) spondylolisthesis. (Illustrated by Jeff Telemeco.)

also used for chronic LBP patients in whom instability is believed to be the cause of pain and fusion the definitive procedure to correct that malady. Similarly, patients with a failed back surgery may undergo fusion if the surgeon feels that instability was created by the prior surgery. Fusion may be performed for some patients having disc degeneration, assuming that disc degeneration equates with spinal instability. Deyo et al. reported that "despite these theories, there is little consensus as to appropriate diagnostic criteria for instability or indications for lumbar spinal fusion."[60]

Spondylolisthesis

Many clinicians attempt to categorize spinal instability through diagnostic tests such as radiographs. A general definition of spinal instability is loss of tissue stiffness resulting in an abnormal increase in joint deformation when a load is applied.[5,61] Given this broad definition, any structural defect of the lumbar spine caused by injury or degeneration may predispose an individual to segmental instability. Conditions that may lead to instability include disc herniation, degenerative disc disease, osteoarthritis, spondylolysis, and spondylolisthesis.[5,62]

Spondylolisthesis is defined as "the forward displacement of one vertebra on another"[63] (Figure 7-6). Various types of spondylolistheses are discussed in Chapter 2. "Despite a wide array of surgical options available, nonoperative care continues to be the mainstay and initial focus of treatment for the adult with isthmic spondylolisthesis."[63] A study by Frennered et al. found that 83% of young patients with symptomatic low-grade slips had excellent or good results at a 7-year follow-up after nonoperative treatment.[64] In the adult population, conservative care that includes trunk strengthening exercises produces favorable results.[65]

Surgical intervention becomes a consideration in those patients with intractable back or leg pain, neurologic signs, cauda equina involvement, and progressive slipping.[63,66] Spinal nerve root decompression or fusion are the available surgical options.[63]

Fusion success rates among adults treated for spondylolisthesis range from 67% to 95%.[67,68] Kim et al. reported 87% of patients with a solid arthrodesis had good or excellent results.[68] Failed fusion leads to an unsatisfactory result in a high percentage of patients.[68,69]

Postoperative Instability

The study of instability related to lumbar surgical procedures is prolific. Sienkiewicz and Flatley reported that laminectomies at multiple levels increased the risk for postoperative spondylolisthesis.[70] Shenkin and Hash reported that spondylolisthesis developed in 15% of patients who underwent bilateral laminectomies and facetectomies of three or more levels, whereas only 6% of patients with removal of two levels demonstrated vertebral slippage.[71] In contrast, Lee reported that laminectomies at multiple levels did not increase the risk for developing spondylolisthesis.[72] Research on cadaveric spinal units revealed better stability during biomechanical testing after internal laminoplasty compared with procedures that involved increased bone resection such as laminectomy, hemilaminectomy, and partial facetectomy.[73] Despite conflicting information, surgeons are performing procedures that minimize bone resection to decrease the possibility of segmental instability.[73,74] Research regarding postoperative instability and clinical outcomes does not support some surgeons' bias that fusion should accompany spinal decompression.[70–72,75]

Instability Secondary to Disc Degeneration

It has been a long-held belief that degenerative disc disease creates instability. Kirkaldy-Willis and Farfan[5] defined increased spinal motion as being excessive range of motion or increased motion in an abnormal direction. They hypothesized that disc disease in the early stages, before significant disc space narrowing and scarring, leads to increased motion, which results in instability. Gertzbein et al.,[76] analyzing instantaneous centers of rotation at the L4–L5 motion segments in cadaver specimens, demonstrated that in the early stages of degeneration, erratic motion (slightly increased translational and rotational motion) was the major abnormality rather than excessive motion (increased range of motion). By the time noticeable disc space narrowing was evident radiographically, the motion segment had stabilized.[76] This suggests that radiographic evidence of degenerative disc disease may be inadequate evidence of the need to perform spinal fusion.

Outcomes of Fusion

Comparing 1,524 Medicare patients undergoing lumbar fusion at one or more segments with Medicare patients undergoing other types of spinal surgery, Deyo et al. found that for those who underwent fusion, the hospitalization time was twice as long, the blood transfusion rate was 3.7 times as high, the mortality was twice as high, nursing home placements were twice as high, and the likelihood of future operations was unchanged.[60] The authors stated that their "data suggest an urgent need for uniform definition of spinal instability and the indications for lumbar spinal fusion."[60]

The difficulty in evaluating the fusion literature is related as much to the surgery performed as it is to the outcomes measured. Typically, reported outcomes lack uniform functional measures on which to evaluate success. Overall, studies report good or excellent results that vary between 39% and 80%, with poor results ranging from 6% to 100%.[77-80] The authors of many studies collectively report a variety of reasons for poor results, including a workers' compensation claim, patients' being out of work for 6 months or longer before surgery, multilevel fusions, smoking, osteoporosis, radiographic pseudarthrosis, poor criterion by which segmental instability is defined, the decision to perform surgery based on discography alone, and the full range of psychosocial barriers. Ironically, the presence of chronic pain is often one of the indications for this procedure, and therefore rehabilitation strategies for most spinal fusion patients should include those outlined in Chapter 5. There is consensus that a solid fusion leads to a better result than does a recurrent pseudarthrosis.[81,82]

Rehabilitation After Fusion

Ideally, the physical therapist plays a key role before surgery. The physical therapist should work in conjunction with the surgeon to determine who is a satisfactory candidate for fusion surgery based on criteria previously reported.

Postsurgically, physical therapists traditionally have limited involvement in the immediate care of spinal fusion patients. Other than assisting in ambulation, demonstrating basic conditioning activities, and educating the patient about how to pursue activities, spinal exercises are not introduced. The principal concern after spinal fusion must be to avoid those activities that could lead to pseudarthrosis. The use of nonsteroidal anti-inflammatory medications is avoided for this reason.[21]

Above the fusion sites, intradiscal pressures in cadavers increased substantially with flexion, and the increase was much greater with two-level fusions. Because of these findings, Weinhoffer et al. recommended limiting spinal flexion.[83] Additionally, the patient's ability to resume normal activities is significantly delayed because of the need to develop a fused mass. Studies by Johnsson et al. demonstrated that the use of a rigid orthosis for 5 months was superior to only 3 months' use among noninstrumented fusion patients in developing a more stable fusion.[84] Childs and Andersson used a rigid orthosis for up to 6 months because of the need to develop a solid fusion mass.[21] They noted that the orthosis cannot prevent intervertebral motions but it does reduce gross motion and the overall load on the spine. They also stated that "the risk of bony failure at the attachment sites for the instrumentation (screws, hooks, and so on) increases rapidly as the bone becomes more osteoporotic. Further, the risk of failure above the instrumented level is also great due to increased stress concentration on the segment adjacent to the rigidly instrumented level."[21] The authors stated that the use of a lumbar orthosis for spinal fusion remains controversial, and in our clinical practice, I find they are rarely used.

Interestingly, the levels above the fusion do not become hypermobile as had previously been assumed. Luk concluded that motion in the adjacent two motion segments above the fusion segments, whether one or two vertebrae were fused, remained hypomobile 5–7 years after the surgery.[85] When considering the problem of degenerative changes at adjacent segments, diminished mobility may be one cause of those changes. This study certainly promotes the need to mobilize the spine after fusion; however, the need to establish a fused mass opposes motion.

With these data seemingly in opposition to good long-term outcomes, the following discussion of rehabilitation will blend what is known with what seems reasonable, and we will wait for data that guide us in a different direction. The rehabilitation guidelines given are under relatively ideal circumstances. For long-term spinal health, the best interests of the patient and the insurance industry are served by a protracted course of rehabilitation.

Table 7-7 gives a temporal summary of intervention beginning presurgically and progressing through 12 months. As with many treatment protocols, the time varies based on the referring surgeon, the patient, and the needs of the situation. It is difficult to defend a protocol without a randomized, double-blind study. The arguments for the protocol are driven by the need to obtain a solid fusion while also meeting the long-term need to mobilize the spine, regain trunk strength, and regain dynamic stability. The guidelines presented in Table 7-7 assume a rigidly instrumented fusion is performed across one or more segments. For patients undergoing a nonin-

Table 7-7 Rehabilitation Guidelines for Patients with Rigidly Instrumented Lumbar Fusions

Rehabilitation strategies	Time after surgery							
	Pre-surgery	0–1 mos	2–4 mos	4–5 mos	5–6 mos	6–9 mos	9–12 mos	12 + mos
Education	■							
Proper body mechanics	■							
Ice		■	■	■				
Walking		■	■	■	■	■	■	
Lower extremity strengthening without lumbar flexion or extension		■	■					
Upper extremity strengthening without flexion or extension			■					
Isometric abdominal exercises			■					
Isometric extension			■					
Soft tissue mobilization			■	■	■			
Quadruped flexion				■	■			
Seated flexion					■			
Hyperextension				■	■	■	■	■
Standing forward bending (unweighted)					■			
Standing lateral flexion (unweighted progressing to weighted)						■	■	■
Seated trunk rotation without lumbar movement					■	■	■	
Weighted forward bending						■	■	■

Rehabilitation strategies	Time after surgery							
	Pre-surgery	0–1 mos	2–4 mos	4–5 mos	5–6 mos	6–9 mos	9–12 mos	12 + mos
Crunches and obliques (obliques not to be started until 6 mos after surgery)								
Unrestricted exercise as tolerated								
Work simulation								

strumented fusion, the guidelines for all movement-related exercises are generally delayed by approximately 2 months. Some spinal surgeons are performing newer techniques that they believe allow them to mobilize the patient earlier. The debate over when to begin movement and which exercise to use is probably analogous to the debate seen with the introduction of newer anterior cruciate ligament reconstruction procedures. Because research cannot keep up with clinical advances, the decisions made by all parties should be carefully considered when faced with little support in the literature.

Forward-bending activities do not begin until the fifth month; however, quadruped flexion begins at 4 months. (In patients with a noninstrumented fusion, quadruped flexion begins at 6 months.) After initiating quadruped flexion, the patient's pain level usually decreases. At 5 months, seated forward bending is permitted and when the patient is well coordinated and comfortable, I start the patient with standing forward bending through limited ranges. Full-range standing forward bending is permitted by the sixth month if this motion is comfortable and well controlled. Beyond 6 months, progression of the patient's exercise program is largely determined by pain tolerance and the presence of a fused mass. The rehabilitation program from this time forward varies in intensity based on the desired goal. If the patient being rehabilitated will be returning to work as a medium to heavy laborer, the ability to engage in that job will be dependent on overall strength and endurance as well as a successful fusion. Few in this job category ever achieve the goal of returning to their former work level.

Most patients who undergo spinal fusion ultimately have the surgery by default. Other treatments have been unsuccessful, and therefore the procedure is typically performed well past the 6-month warning mark for chronic pain. Although there are a few exceptions, generally consider a spinal fusion patient as a chronic pain patient. After an initial assessment, if there appear to be no barriers to recovery and symptom magnification is not an issue, the possibility of problems arising later is still substantial, since the postoperative recovery after a fusion is protracted and painful. The first 4 months are particularly difficult, largely because of bone pain. By 5 months, pain is typically lower than it was preoperatively, walking is comfortable, and the activity level is much higher.

In our office, many patients who have a spinal fusion do return to gainful employment but usually with some modifications, unless their jobs were light or sedentary. For older adults, I remind the patient that a lumbar fusion is a difficult procedure from which to recover. The final goal is a reduction in pain and a return to normal activities. Patients should avoid activities such as golf altogether. Performing activities around the house such as gardening is a realistic goal when performed with minor modifications. The patient should anticipate, under most circumstances, to be able to walk essentially unlimited distances and sit comfortably for long periods with little discomfort.

The reality in clinical practice is that most patients have not received adequate instruction before surgery and expect a complete resolution of symptoms. Whether this is the result of poor preparation on the part of the surgeon or a general expectation that surgery is the ultimate answer, patients are usually disappointed. Patients are usually referred for rehabilitation at least 2 months after surgery and are frustrated that their activity level is very low, that their pain level is very high, and that they are unexpectedly faced with a permanent restriction in activity level. Often the surgeon is encouraging the patient to return faster than the research supports. As stated previously, such patients usually are not wearing a rigid orthosis, they typically smoke, they do not comply with instructions to limit forward bending, and they deny the very real possibility that their outcome may be less than satisfactory. Consequently, treatment of spinal fusion patients should be undertaken only when the physical therapist has trained under someone with experience treating spinal fusion patients and has a full understanding of the available literature, the implementation of a reasonable protocol, and a good working relationship with the referring surgeon.

Conclusion

If research has stoked the fires of debate regarding the efficacy of surgery for LBP, the lack of research on postoperative lumbar rehabilitation has seemingly gone unnoticed. Research fortunately has begun to highlight the need for postoperative lumbar rehabilitation, and its efficacy is being studied. At a time in which cost containment and outcome studies are closely scrutinized, the literature is clear for postsurgical rehabilitation candidates: Therapy must be of adequate duration and intensity to achieve maximum results. Many factors can delay a patient's progression. In the long run, everyone's best interests are served by continuing treatment until all parties are satisfied that maximum improvement has been achieved. If the patient is satisfied that the best possible outcome has been achieved, future costs for that patient's care are likely to be much less than if, at the end of rehabilitation, the patient is continuing to seek a cure. Case workers and mental health professionals can help bring consensus among health care professionals and patients regarding the acceptance of some physical limitations and even the presence of pain as being the best possible outcome. Patients need to understand that surgery for lumbar disorders has specific purposes but is not a cure. Although a specific condition that created pain may have been surgically altered, the disc is still unhealthy, nerve damage may be irreparable, a spondylolisthesis—although stabilized—remains an abnormality, and spinal trauma from the surgery itself can cause problems. For these reasons and many more, patient education remains a high priority and should be the starting point for all rehabilitation programs.

References

1. Mixter WJ, Barr JS. Rupture of the intervertebral disc with involvement of the spinal canal. N Engl J Med 1934;211:210.
2. Anderson R. Diagnosis and Treatment of Low Back Pain Since 1850. In AH White, R Anderson (eds), Conservative Care of Low Back Pain. Baltimore: Williams & Wilkins, 1991;8.
3. Cherkin DC, Deyo RA, Loeser JD, et al. An international comparison of back surgery rates. Spine 1994;19:1201.
4. McNab I. The traction spur: an indicator of segmental instability. J Bone Joint Surg Am 1971;53:663.
5. Kirkaldy-Willis WH, Farfan HF. Instability of lumbar spine. Clin Orthop 1982;165:110.
6. Saal JA, Saal JS, Herzog RJ. The natural history of lumbar intervertebral disc extrusions treated nonoperatively. Spine 1990;15:683.
7. Long DM. Failed back surgery syndrome. Neurosurg Clin North Am 1991;2:899.
8. Junge A, Dvorak J, Ahrens S. The predictors of bad and good outcomes of lumbar disc surgery: prospective clinical study with recommendations for screening to avoid bad outcomes. Spine 1995;20:460.

9. Manniche C, Skall HF, Braendholdt L, et al. Clinical trial of postoperative dynamic back exercises after first lumbar discectomy. Spine 1993;18:92.

10. Manniche C, Asmussen K, Lauritsen B, et al. Intensive dynamic back exercises with or without hyperextension in chronic back pain after surgery for lumbar disc protrusion. Spine 1993;18:560.

11. Manniche C. Assessment and exercise in low back pain: with special reference to the management of pain and disability following the first time lumbar surgery. Dan Med Bull 1995;42:301.

12. Timm KE. A randomized-control study of active and passive treatments for chronic low back pain following L5 laminectomy. J Orthop Sports Phys Ther 1994;20:276.

13. Timm KE. Case Report: Use of Trunk Dynamometers in the Management of Patients with Spinal Disorders. In BP D'Orazio (ed), Back Pain Rehabilitation. Boston: Andover Medical Publishers, 1993;238.

14. Kahanovitz N, Viola K, Gallagher M. Long-term strength assessment of postoperative discectomy patients. Spine 1989;14:402.

15. Rantanen J, Hurme M, Falck B, et al. The lumbar multifidus muscle five years after surgery for a lumbar intervertebral disc herniation. Spine 1993;18:568.

16. Young S, Veerapen R, O'Laorre SA. Relief of lumbar canal stenosis using multilevel subarticular fenestrations as an alternative to wide laminectomy: a preliminary report. Neurosurgery 1988;23:628.

17. Bookwalter JW, Busch MD, Nicely D. Ambulatory surgery is safe and effective in radicular disc disease. Spine 1994;19:526.

18. Epstein NE, Epstein JA, Carras R, Hyman RA. Far lateral lumbar disc herniations and associated structural abnormalities. Spine 1990;15:534.

19. Epstein NE. Evaluation of varied surgical approaches used in the management of 170 far-lateral lumbar disc herniations: indications and results. J Neurosurg 1995;83:648.

20. Hardy MA. The biology of scar formation. Phys Ther 1989;69:1014.

21. Childs RC, Andersson GBJ. Rehabilitation After Back Surgery. In BP D'Orazio (ed), Back Pain Rehabilitation. Boston: Andover Medical Publishers, 1993;72.

22. Matsui H, Kitagawa H, Kawaguchi Y, Tsuji H. Physiologic changes of nerve root during posterior lumbar discectomy. Spine 1995;20:654.

23. Sihvonen T, Herno A, Paljarvi L, et al. Local denervation atrophy of paraspinal muscles in postoperative failed back syndrome. Spine 1993;18:575.

24. Annertz M, Jonsson B, Stromqvist B, Holtas S. No relationship between epidural fibrosis and sciatica in the lumbar postdiscectomy syndrome. Spine 1995;20:449.

25. Fraser RD, Sandhu A, Gogan WJ. Magnetic resonance imaging findings 10 years after treatment for lumbar disc herniation. Spine 1995;20:710.

26. Jensen TT, Overgaard S, Thomsen N, et al. Postoperative computed tomography three months after lumbar disc surgery: a prospective single blind study. Spine 1991;16:620.

27. Smith SA, Massie JB, Chesnut R, Garfin SR. Straight leg raising: anatomical effects on the spinal nerve root with and without fusion. Spine 1993;18:992.

28. Hasue M. Pain and the nerve root: an interdisciplinary approach. Spine 1993;18:2053.

29. Naftulin S, Fast A, Thomas M. Diabetic lumbar radiculopathy: sciatica without disc herniation. Spine 1993;18:2419.

30. Crenshaw AH (ed). Campbell's Operative Orthopaedics (8th ed). Baltimore: Mosby–Year Book, 1992;5.

31. Fernyhough JC, Schimandle JJ, Weigel MC, et al. Chronic donor site pain complicating graft harvesting from the posterior iliac crest for spinal fusion. Spine 1992;17:1474.

32. Maigne JY, Rime B, Deligne B. Computed tomographic follow-up study of forty-eight of nonoperatively treated lumbar intervertebral disc herniation. Spine 1992;17:1071.

33. Berkson MH. Mechanical properties of the human lumbar spine flexibilities, intradiscal pressures, posterior element influences. Proc Inst Med 1977;31:138.

34. Hirsch C, Nachemson A. A new observation on the mechanical behavior of lumbar discs. Acta Orthop Scand 1954;23:254.

35. Hickey DS, Hukins DWL. Relation between the structure of the annulus fibrosus and the function and failure of the intervertebral disc. Spine 1980;5:106.

36. Holmes AD, Hukins DWL, Freemont AJ. End-plate displacement during compression of lumbar vertebra-disc-vertebra segments and the mechanism of failure. Spine 1993;18:128.

37. Gordon SJ, Yang KH, Mayer PJ, et al. Mechanism of disc rupture: a preliminary report. Spine 1991;16:450.

38. Brant-Zawadzki M, Jensen M. Imaging corner spinal nomenclature. Spine 1995;20:388.

39. Surin VV. Duration of disability following lumbar disc surgery. Acta Orthop Scand 1977;48:466.

40. Atlas SJ, Deyo RA, Keller RB, et al. The Maine Lumbar Spine Study, Part II: 1-year outcomes of sugical and nonsurgical management of sciatica. Spine 1996;21:1777.

41. Postacchini F. Results of surgery compared with conservative management for lumbar disc herniations. Spine 1996;21:1383.

42. Delauche-Cavallier MC, Budet C, Laredo JD, et al. Lumbar disc herniation: computed tomography scan changes after conservative treatment of nerve root compression. Spine 1992;17:927.

43. Weber H. Lumbar disc herniation: controlled prospective study with 10 years of observation. Spine 1983;8:131.

44. Carragee EJ, Helms E, O'Sullivan GS. Are postoperative activity restrictions necessary after posterior lumbar discectomy: a prospective study of outcomes in 50 consecutive cases. Spine 1996;21:1893.

45. Battie MC, Videman T, Gill K, et al. Smoking and lumbar intervertebral disc degeneration: an MRI study of identical twins. Spine 1991;16:1015.

46. Jarvinen P, Aho K. Twin studies in rheumatic diseases. Semin Arthritis Rheum 1994;24:19.

47. An HS, Silveri CP, Simpson M, et al. Comparison of smoking habits between parents with surgically confirmed herniated lumbar and cervical disc disease and controls. J Spinal Disord 1994;7:369.

48. Winston K, Rumbaugh C, Colucci V. The vertebral canals in lumbar disc disease. Spine 1984;9:414.

49. Janjua MZ, Muhammad F. Measurements of the normal adult lumbar spinal canal. J Pak Med Assoc 1989;39:264.

50. Postacchini F, Pezzeri G, Montanaro A, Natali G. Computerized tomography in lumbar stenosis. J Bone Joint Surg Br 1980;62:78.

51. Takahashi K, Miyazaki T, Takino T, et al. Epidural pressure measurements: relationship between epidural pressure and posture in patients with lumbar spinal stenosis. Spine 1995;20:650.

52. Atlas SJ, Deyo RA, Keller RB, et al. The Maine Lumbar Spine Study, part III: one-year outcomes of surgical and nonsurgical management of lumbar spinal stenosis. Spine 1996;21:1787.

53. Johnsson KE, Uden A, Rosen I. The effect of decompression on the natural course of spinal stenosis: a comparison of surgically treated and untreated patients. Spine 1991;16:615.

54. Herno A, Airaksinen O, Saari T. Long-term results of surgical treatment of lumbar spinal stenosis. Spine 1993;18:1471.

55. Hashimoto M, Watanabe O, Hirano H. Extraforaminal stenosis in the lumbosacral spine: efficacy of MR imaging in the coronal plane. Acta Radiol 1996;37:610.

56. Airaksinen O, Herno A, Turunen V, et al. Surgical outcome of 438 patients treated for lumbar spinal stenosis. Spine 1997;22:2278.

57. Katz JN, Lipson SJ, Brick GW, et al. Clinical correlates of patient satisfaction after laminectomy for degenerative lumbar spinal stenosis. Spine 1995;20:1155.

58. Deen HG, Zimmerman RS, Lyons MK, et al. Measurement of exercise tolerance on the treadmill in patients with symptomatic lumbar spinal atenosis: a useful indicator of functional status and surgical outcome. J Neurosurg 1995;83:27.
59. Amundsen T, Weber H, Lilleas F, et al. Lumbar spinal stenosis: clinical and radiological features. Spine 1995;20:1178.
60. Deyo A, Ciol MA, Cherkin DC, et al. Lumbar spinal fusion: a cohort study of complications, reoperations, and resource use in medicare population. Spine 1993;19:1463.
61. Pope MH, Panjabi M. Biomechanical definitions of spinal instability. Spine 1985;10:255.
62. Morgan FP, King T. Primary instability of lumbar vertebrae as a common cause of low back pain. J Bone Joint Surg Br 1957;39:6.
63. Lauerman WC, Cain JE. Isthmic spondylolisthesis in the adult. J Am Acad Orthop Surg 1996;4:201.
64. Frennered AK, Danielson BI, Nachemson AL. Natural history of symptomatic isthmic low-grade spondylolisthesis in children and adolescents: a seven-year follow-up study. J Ped Orthop 1991;11:209.
65. Sinaki M, Lutness MP, Ilstrup DM, et al. Lumbar spondylolisthesis: retrospective comparison and three-year follow-up of two conservative treatment programs. Arch Phys Med Rehabil 1989;70:594.
66. Bradford DS. Treatment of spondylolysis and spondylolisthesis: dysplastic and lytic lesions in children and adults. Presented at the 61st Annual Meeting of the American Academy of Orthopaedic Surgeons; February 25, 1994; New Orleans, LA.
67. Stauffer RN, Coventry MB. Posterolateral lumbar-spine fusion. J Bone Joint Surg Am 1972;54:1195.
68. Kim SS, Denis F, Lonstein JE, Winter RB. Factors affecting fusion rate in adult spondylolisthesis. Spine 1990;15:979.
69. Hanley EN, Levy JA. Surgical treatment of isthmic lumbosacral spondylolisthesis: of variables influencing results. Spine 1989;14:48.
70. Sienkiewicz PJ, Flatley TJ. Postoperative spondylolisthesis. Clin Orthop 1987;221:172.
71. Shenkin HA, Hash CJ. Spondylolisthesis after multiple bilateral laminectomies and facetectomies for lumbar spondylosis: follow-up review. J Neurosurg 1979;50:45.
72. Lee CK. Lumbar spinal instability (olisthesis) after extensive posterior spinal decompression. Spine 1983;8:429.
73. Efstathiou P, Moskovich R, Casar R, Magnisalis E. A biomedical evaluation of internal lumbar laminoplasty: the preservation of spinal stabil-

ity during laminectomy for degenerative spinal stenosis. Bull Hosp Joint Dis 1996;55:7.

74. Okawa A, Shinomiya K, Takakuda K, Nakai O. A cadaveric study of the stability of lumbar segment after partial laminotomy and facetectomy with intact posterior ligaments. J Spinal Disord 1996;9:518.

75. Johnsson KE, Willner S, Johnsson K. Postoperative instability after decompression for lumbar spinal stenosis. Spine 1986;11:107.

76. Gertzbein SD, Seligman J, Holtby R, et al. Centrode patterns and segmental instability in degenerative disc disease. Spine 1985;10:257.

77. Knox BD, Chapman TM. Anterior lumbar interbody fusion for discogram concordant pain. J Spinal Disord 1993;6:242.

78. Zdeblick TA. The prospective, randomized study of lumbar fusion: preliminary results. Spine 1993;18:983.

79. Parker LM, Murrell SE, Boden SD, Horton WC. The outcome of posterolateral fusion in highly selected patients with discogenic low back pain. Spine 1996;21:1909.

80. Gill K, Blumenthal SL. Functional results after anterior lumbar fusion at L5-S1 in patients with normal and abnormal MRI scans. Spine 1992;17:940.

81. Lauerman WC, Bradford DS. Results of lumbar pseudarthrosis repair. J Spinal Disord 1992;5:149.

82. Kim SS, Michelsen CB. Revision surgery for failed back surgery syndrome. Spine 1992;17:957.

83. Weinhoffer SL, Guyer D, Herbert M, Griffith SL. Intradiscal pressure measurements above an instrumented fusion: a cadaveric study. Spine 1995;20:526.

84. Johnsson R, Stromqvist B, Axelsson P, Selvik G. Influence of spinal immobilization on consolidation of posterolateral lumbosacral fusion: a Roentgen stereophotogrammetric and radiographic analysis. Spine 1992;17:16.

85. Luk KDK, Chow DHK, Evans JH, Leong JCY. Lumbar spinal mobility after short anterior interbody fusion. Spine 1995;20:813.

Index

Note: Page numbers in *italics* refer to illustrations; page numbers followed by t refer to tables.